Baby Shower For

Date

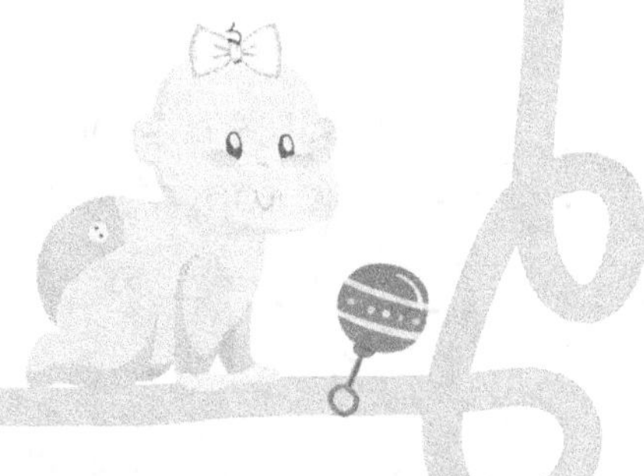

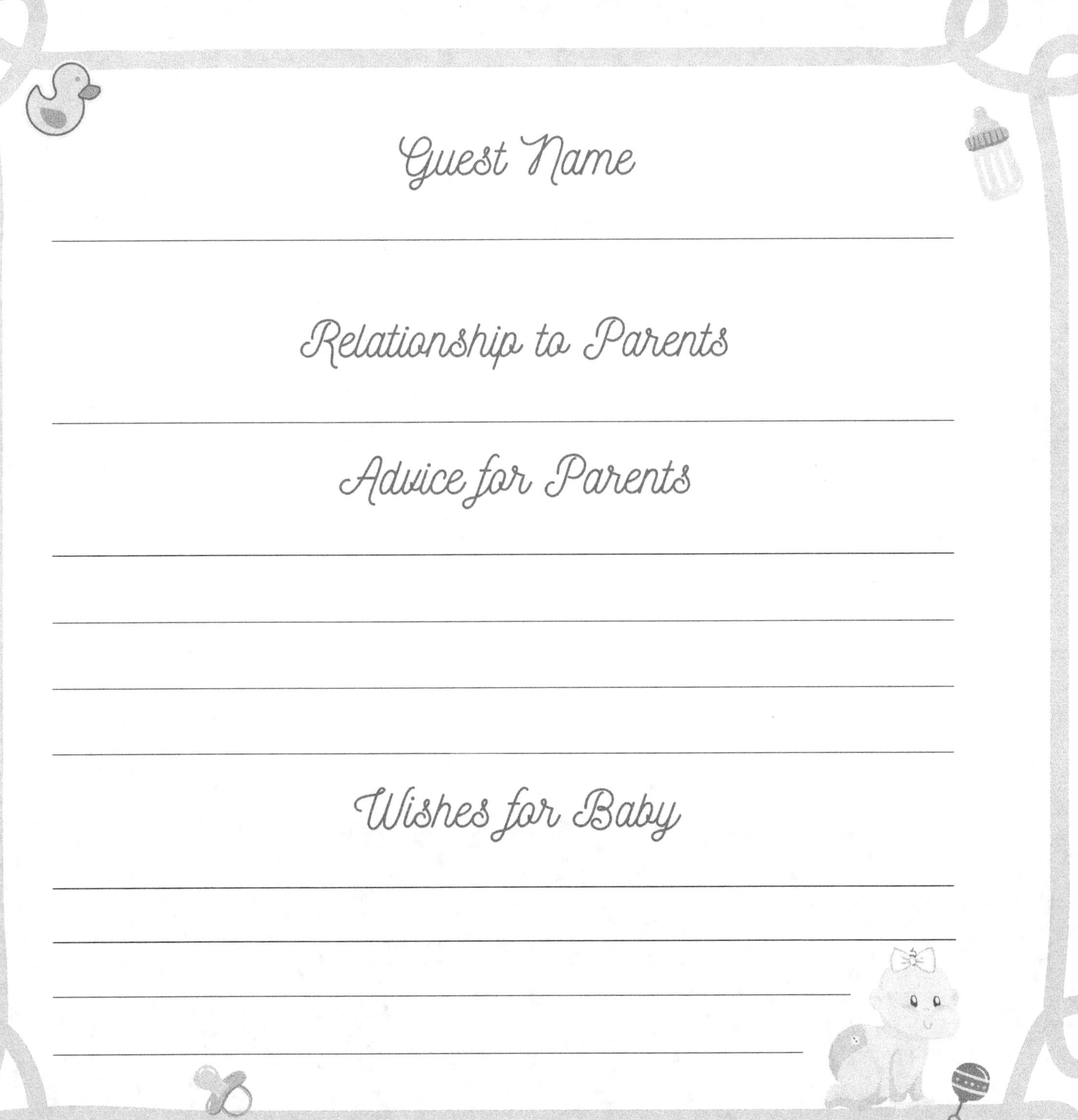

Guest Name

Relationship to Parents

Advice for Parents

Wishes for Baby

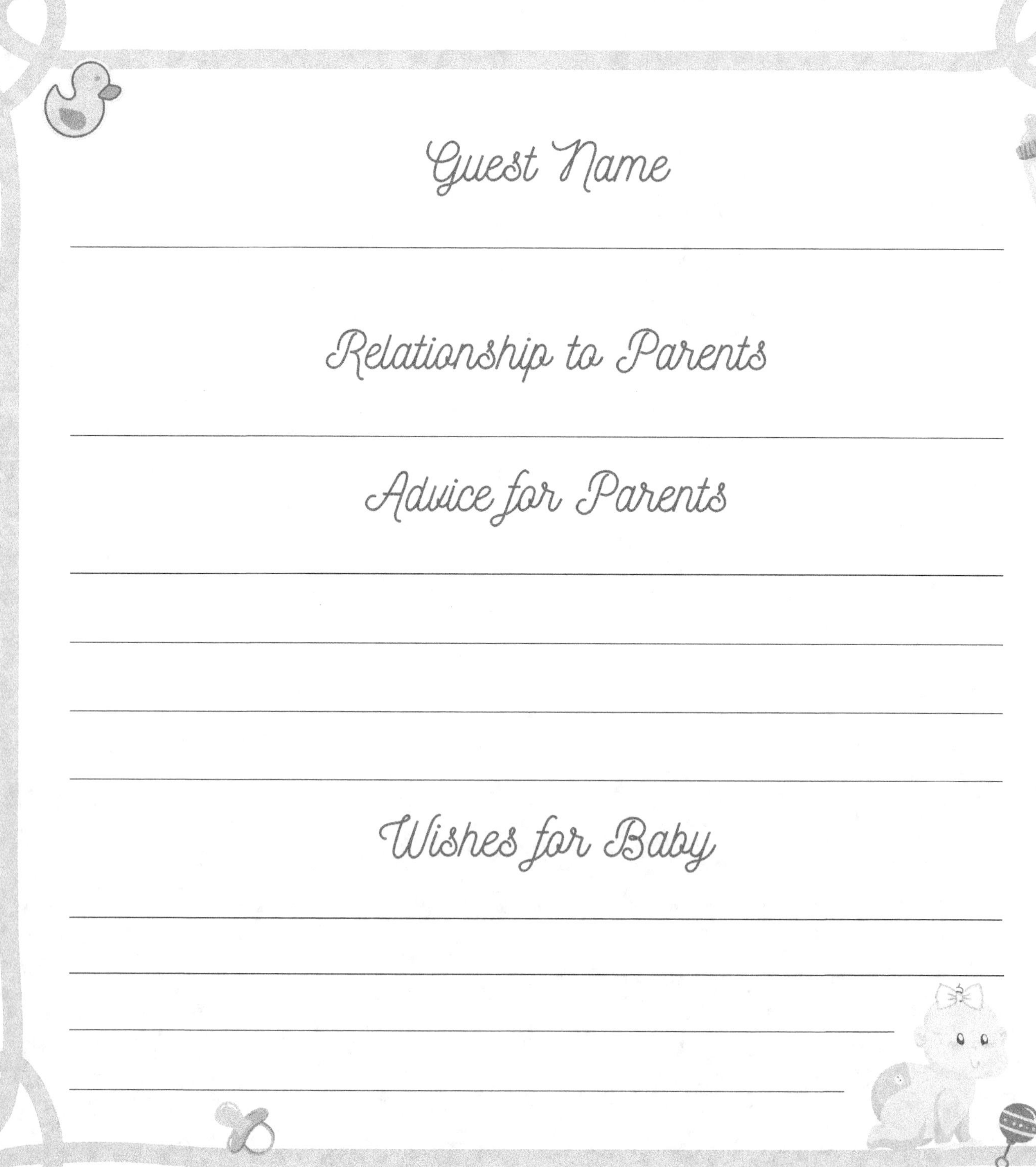

Guest Name

Relationship to Parents

Advice for Parents

Wishes for Baby

Guest Name

Relationship to Parents

Advice for Parents

Wishes for Baby

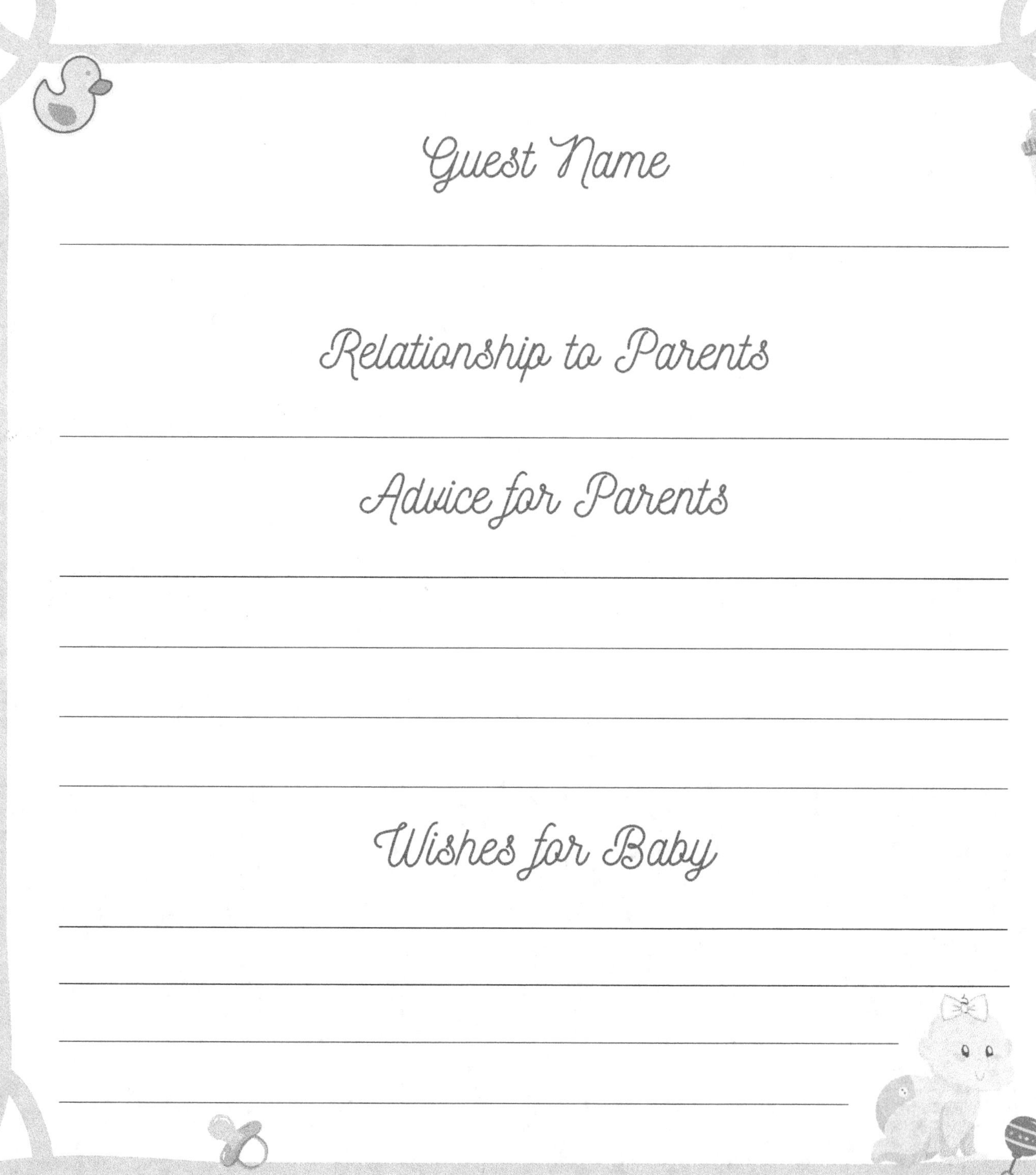

Guest Name

Relationship to Parents

Advice for Parents

Wishes for Baby

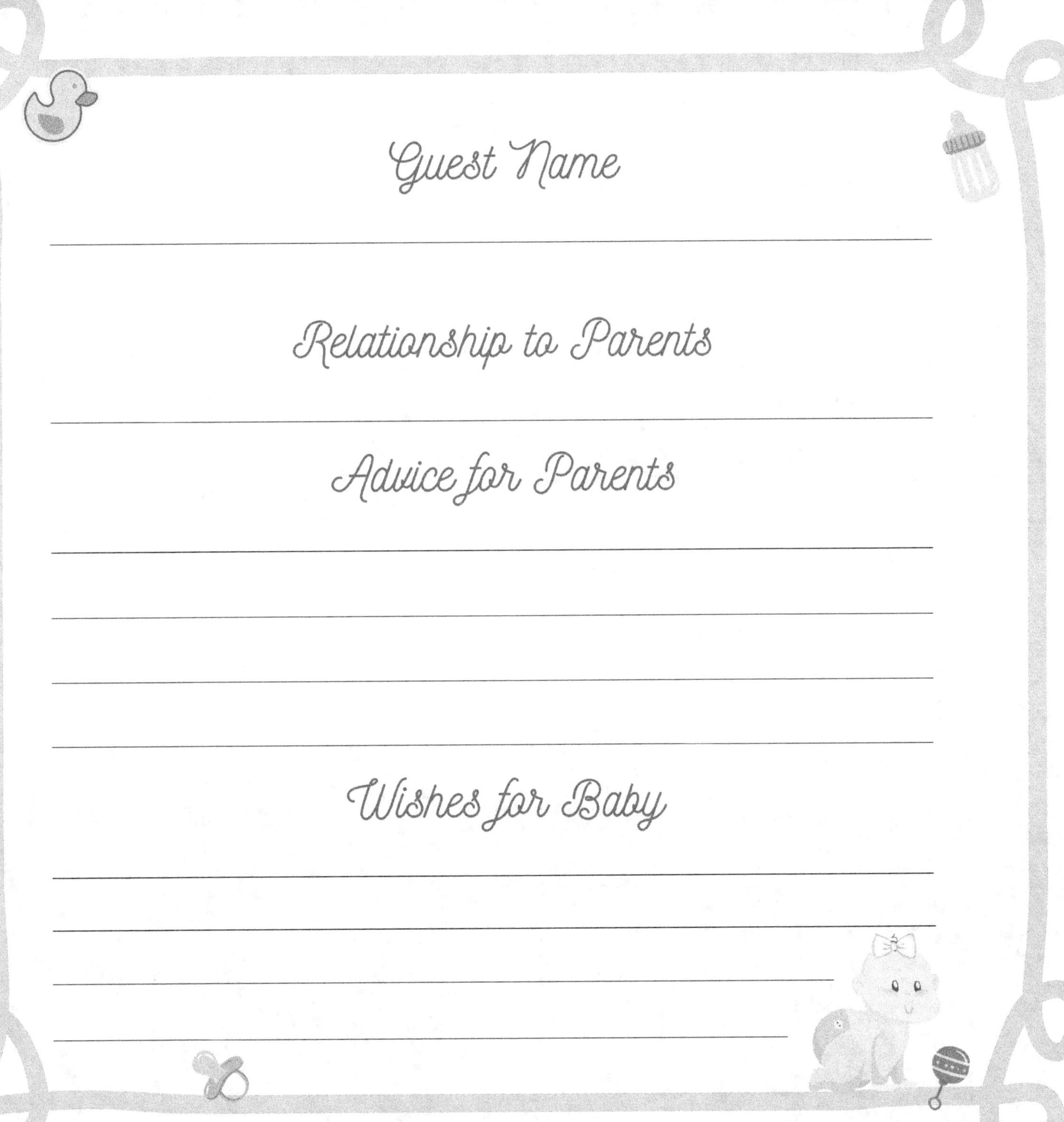
Guest Name
Relationship to Parents
Advice for Parents
Wishes for Baby

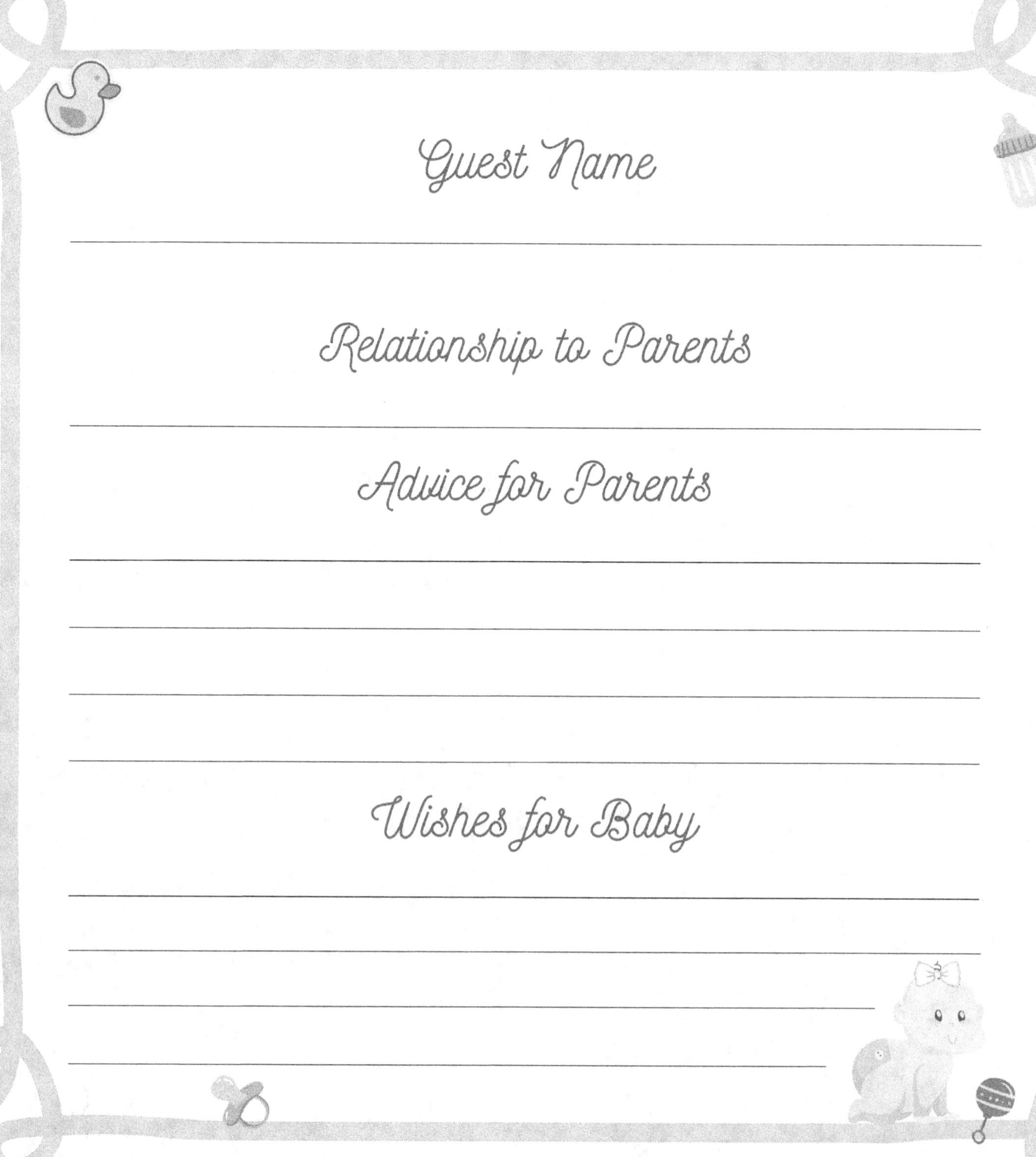

Guest Name
Relationship to Parents
Advice for Parents
Wishes for Baby

Guest Name

Relationship to Parents

Advice for Parents

Wishes for Baby

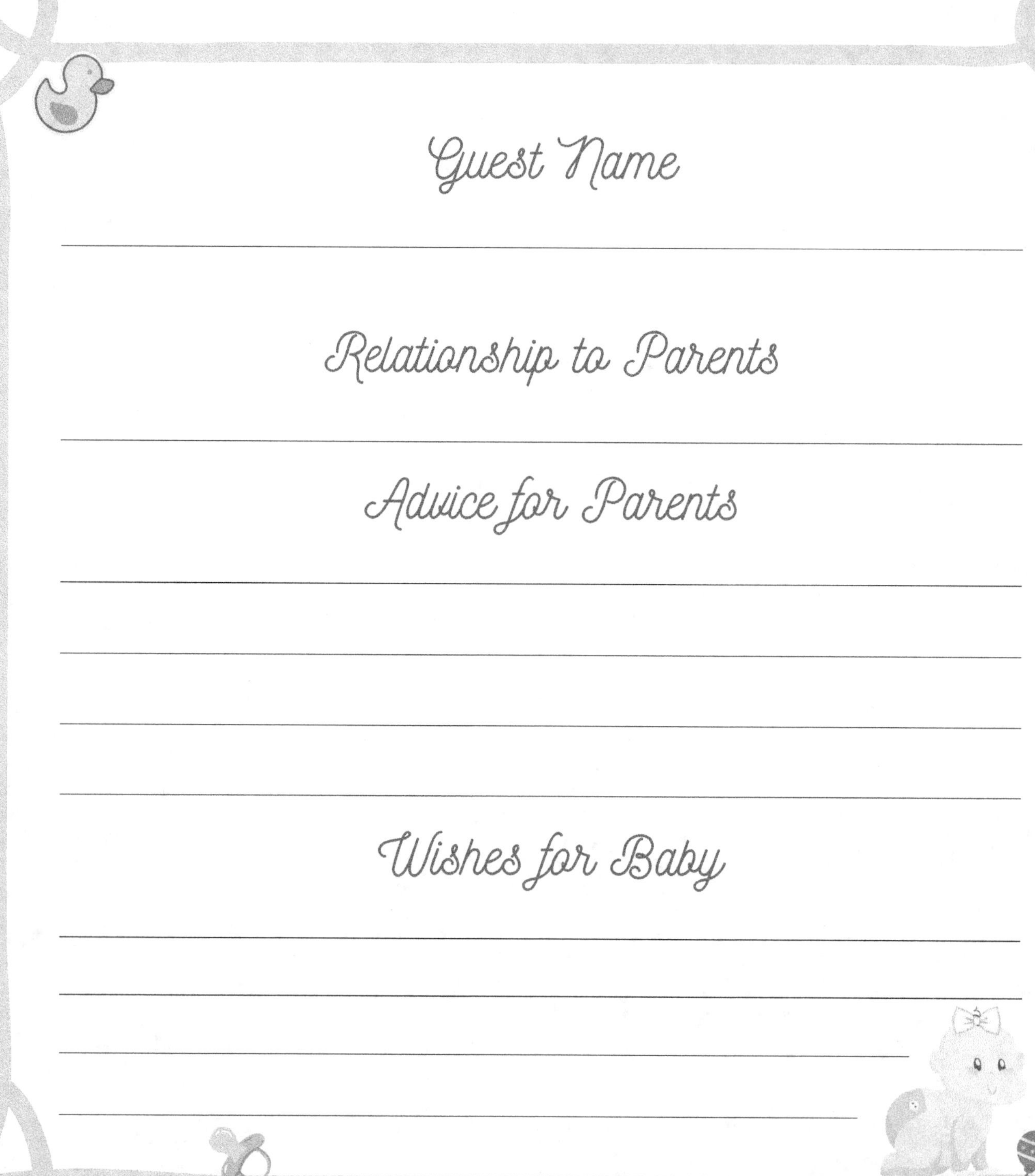

Guest Name

Relationship to Parents

Advice for Parents

Wishes for Baby

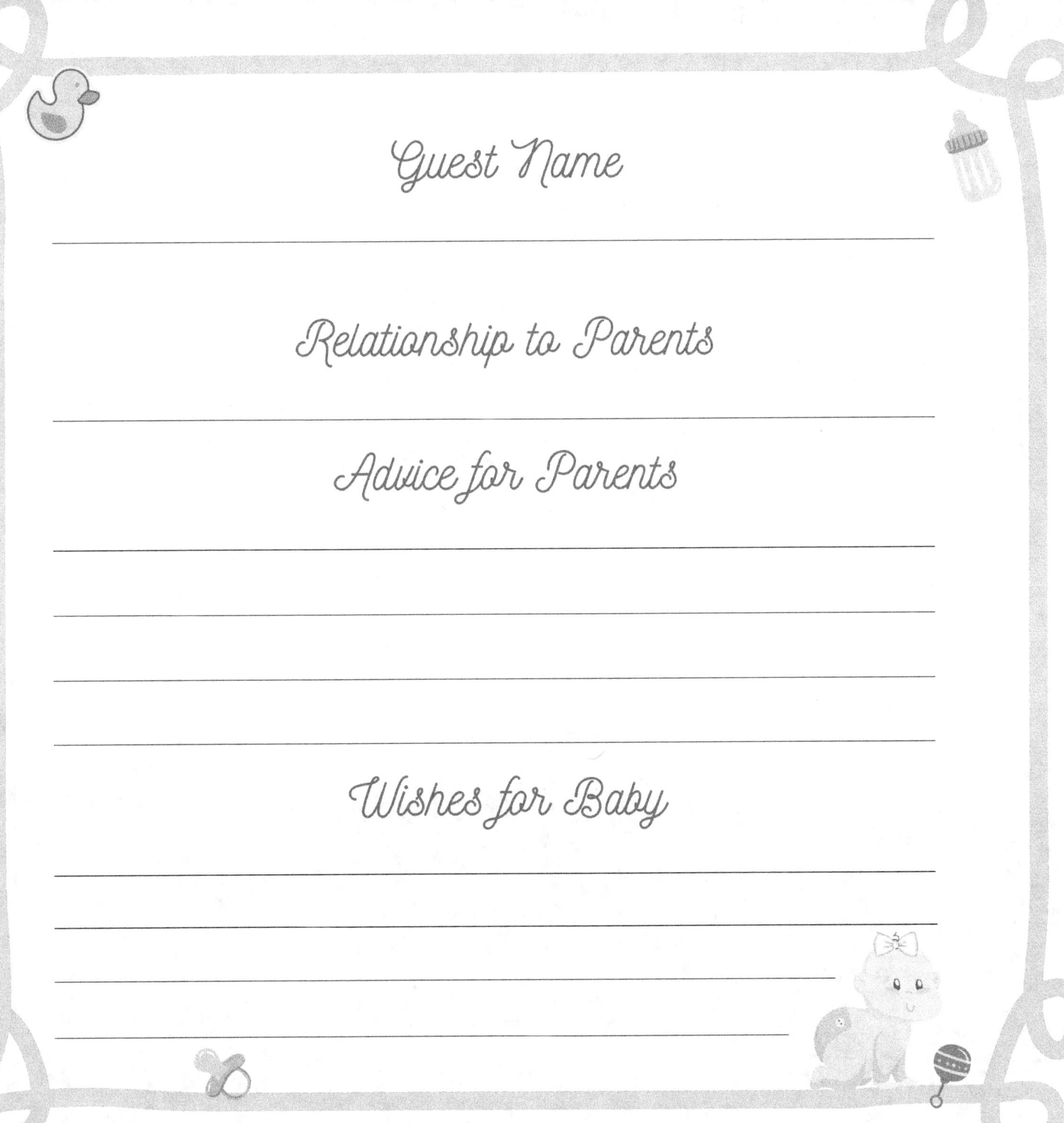

Guest Name
Relationship to Parents
Advice for Parents
Wishes for Baby

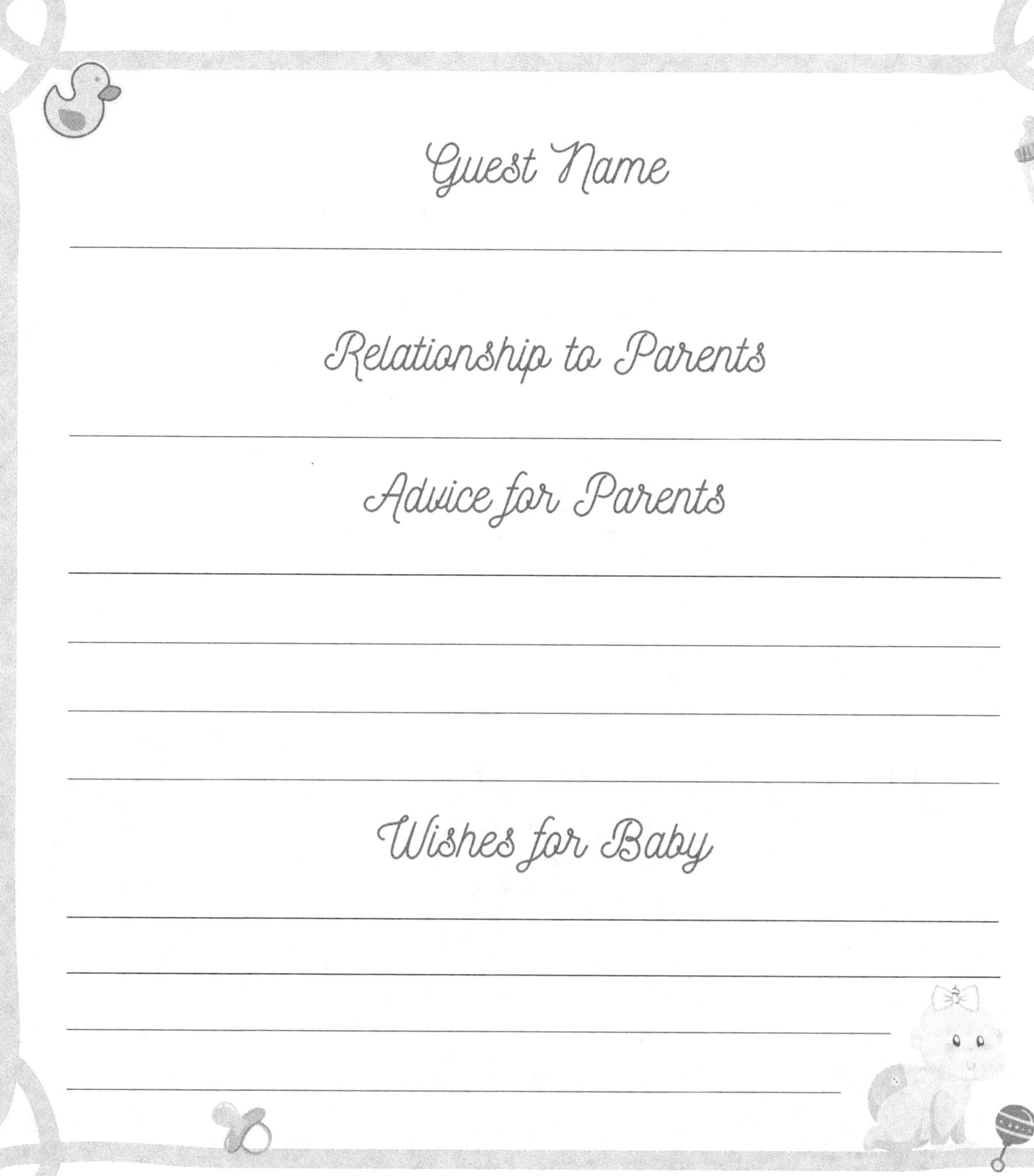
Guest Name
Relationship to Parents
Advice for Parents
Wishes for Baby

Guest Name

Relationship to Parents

Advice for Parents

Wishes for Baby

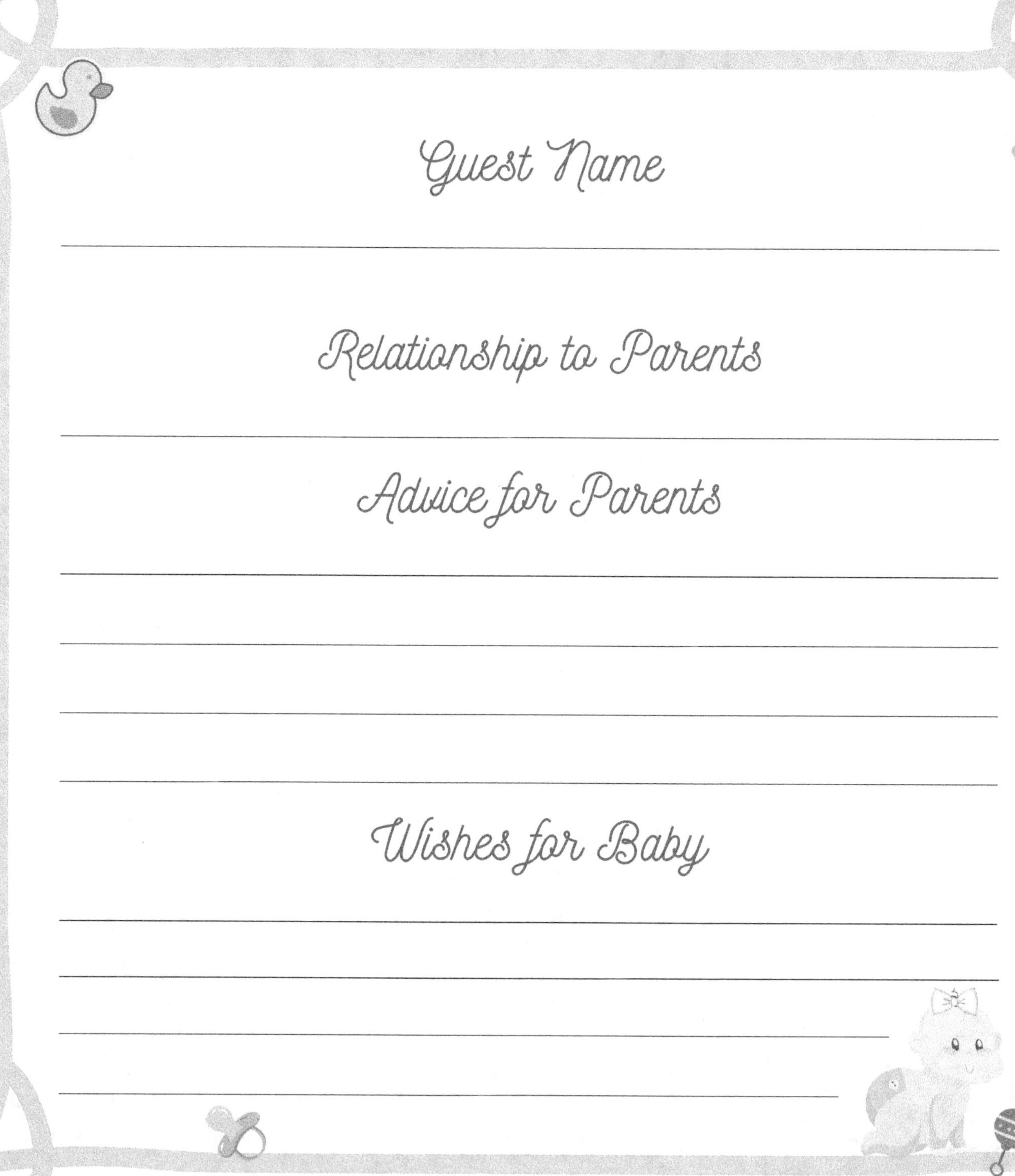

Guest Name

Relationship to Parents

Advice for Parents

Wishes for Baby

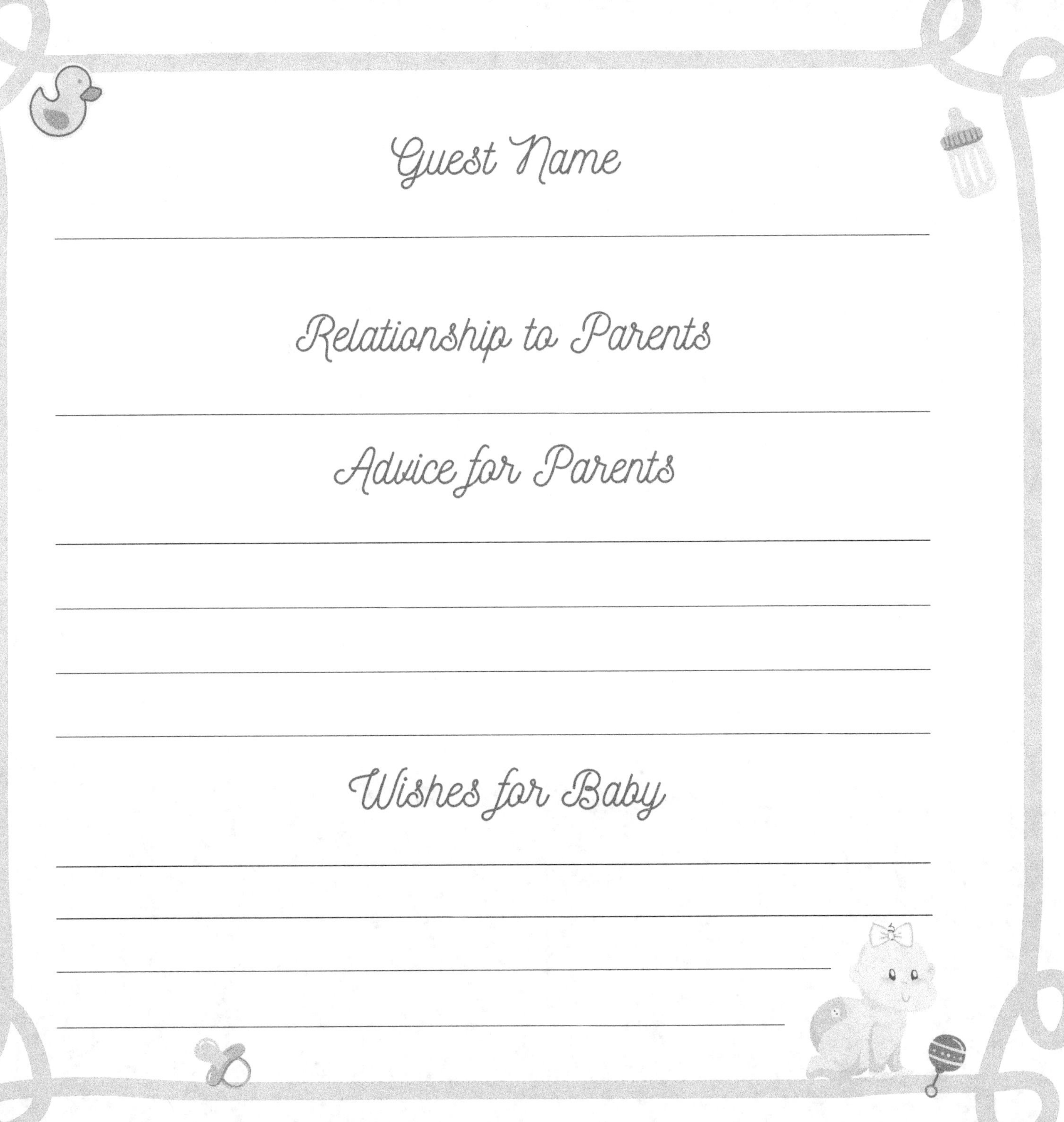
Guest Name
Relationship to Parents
Advice for Parents
Wishes for Baby

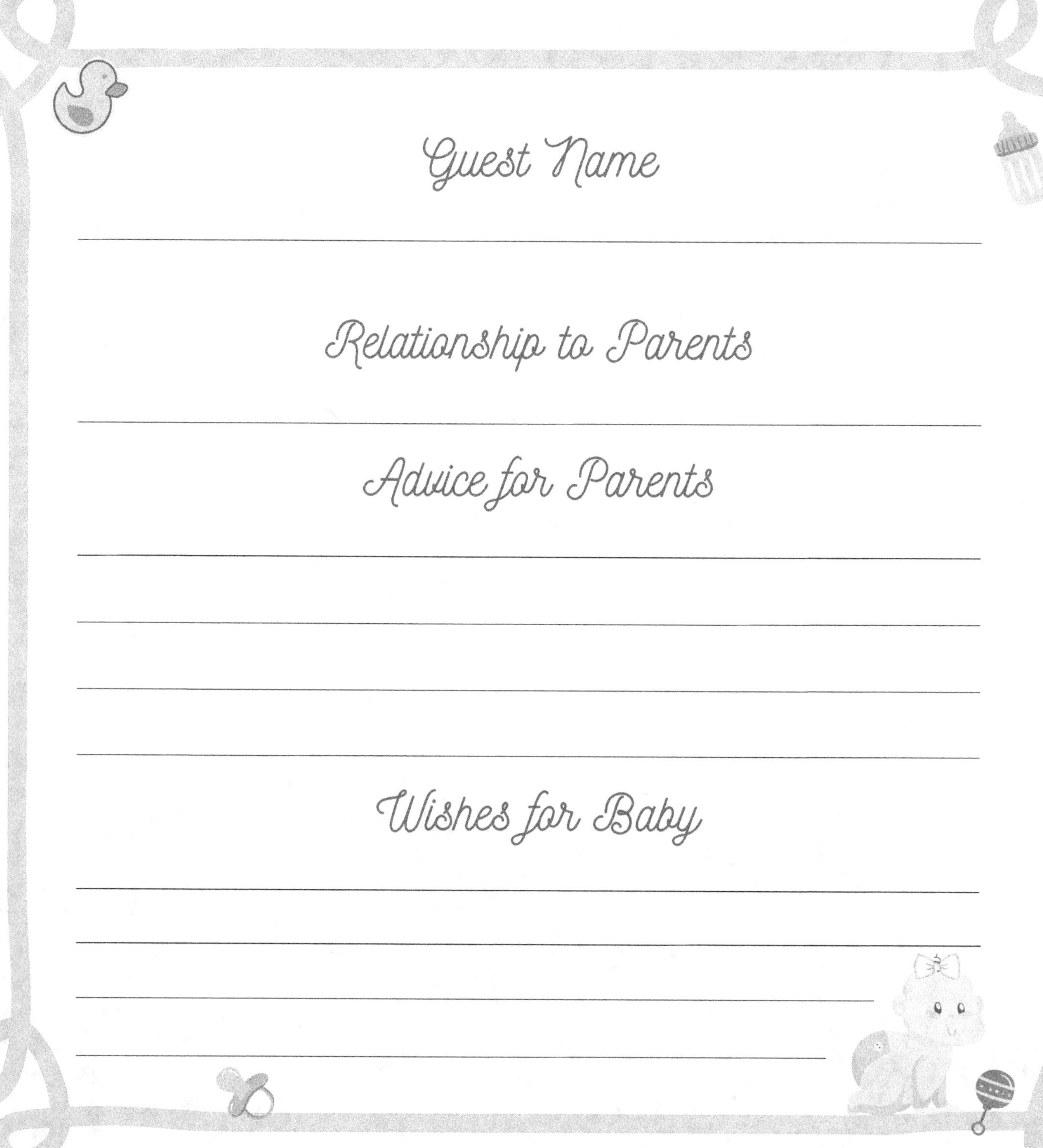
Guest Name

Relationship to Parents

Advice for Parents

Wishes for Baby

Guest Name

Relationship to Parents

Advice for Parents

Wishes for Baby

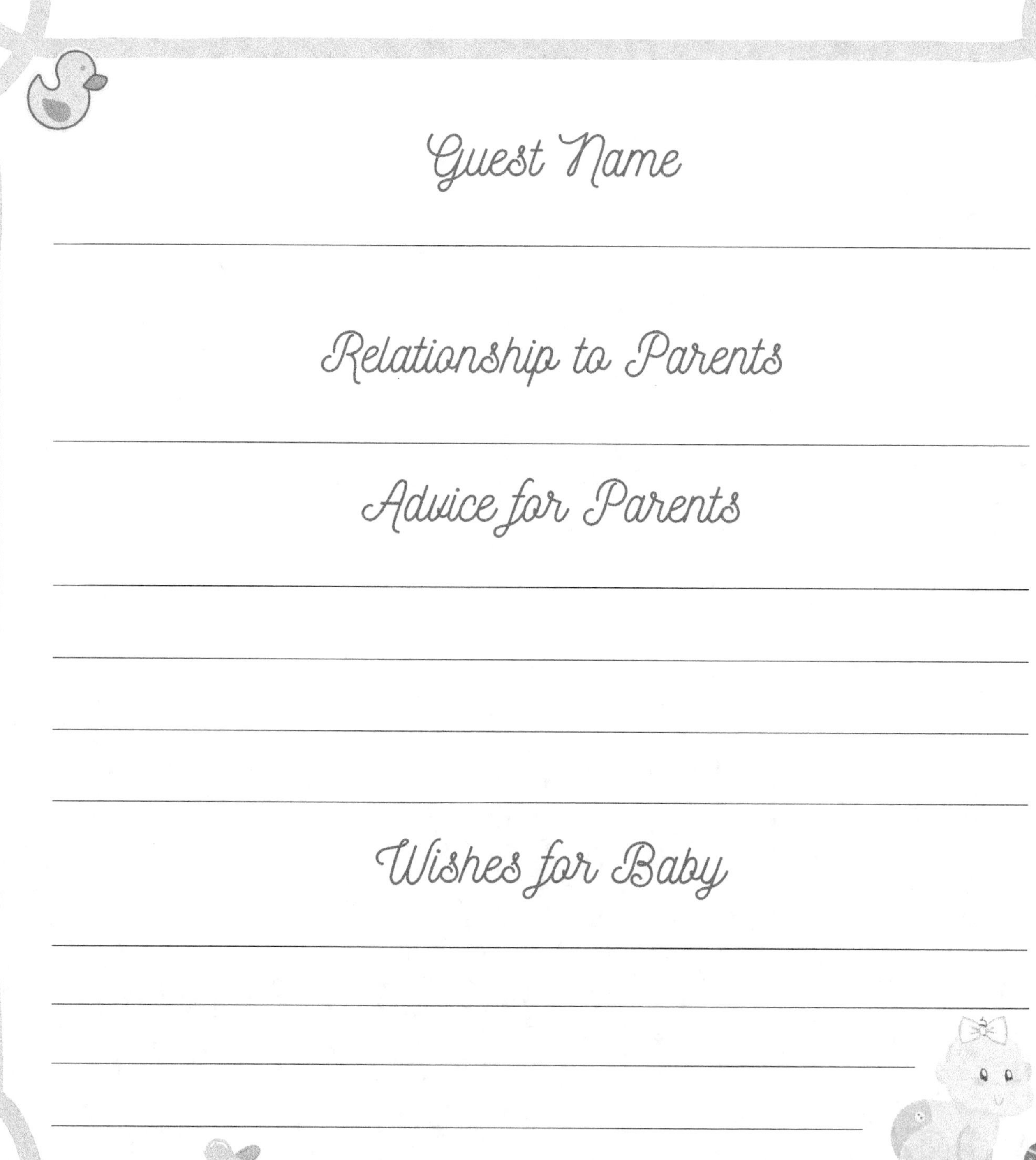

Guest Name

Relationship to Parents

Advice for Parents

Wishes for Baby

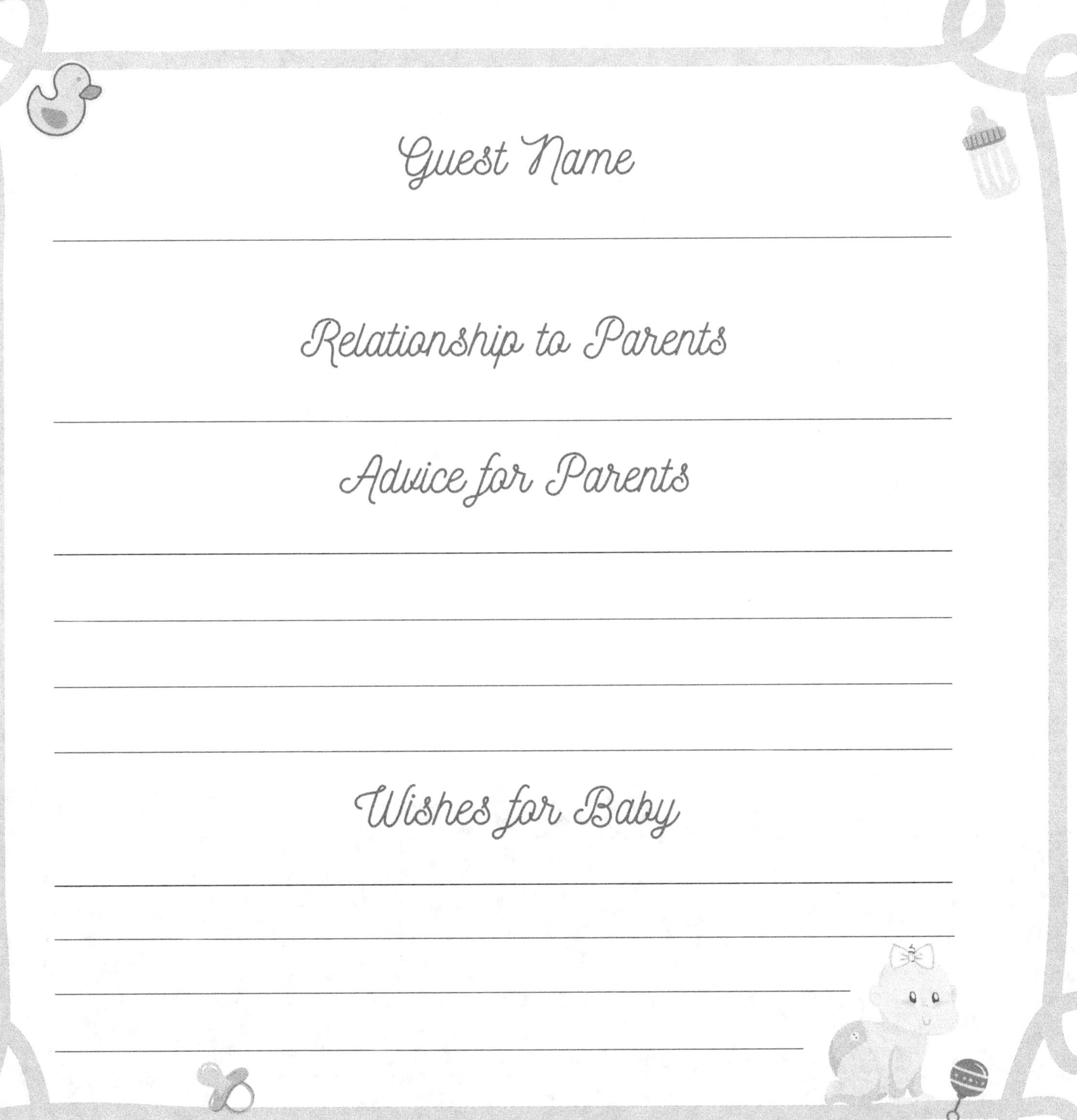

Guest Name

Relationship to Parents

Advice for Parents

Wishes for Baby

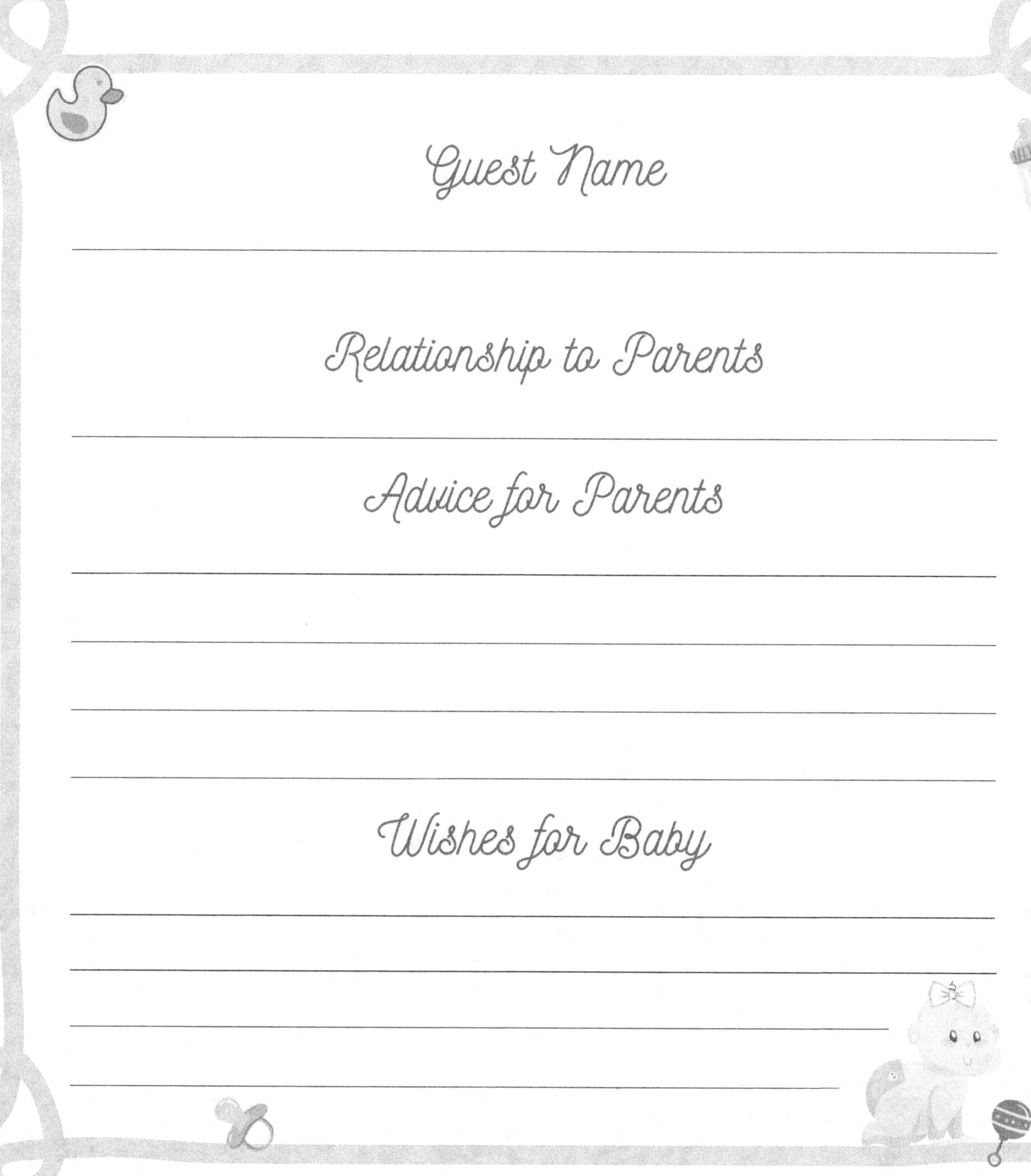
Guest Name

Relationship to Parents

Advice for Parents

Wishes for Baby

Guest Name

Relationship to Parents

Advice for Parents

Wishes for Baby

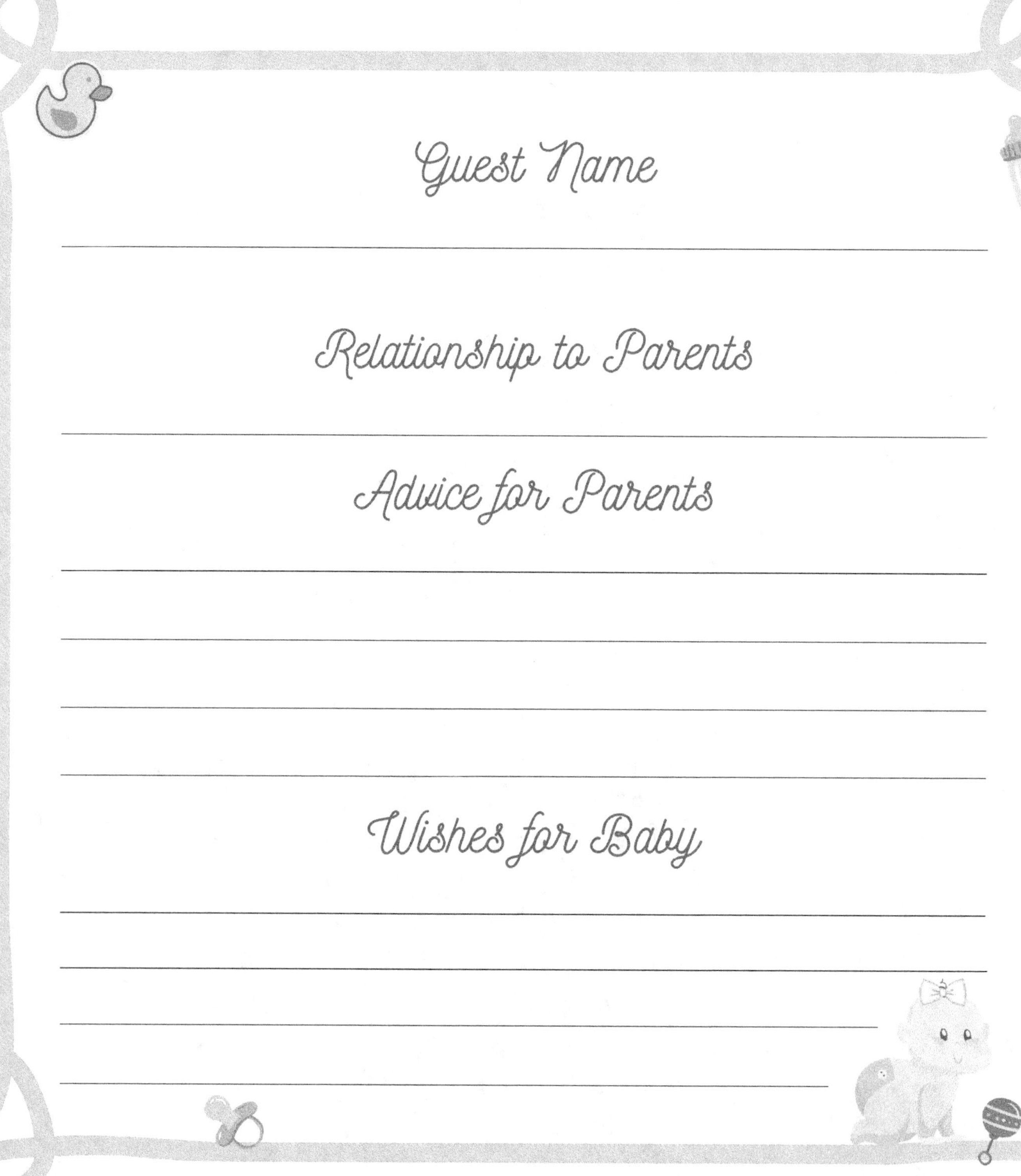
Guest Name

Relationship to Parents

Advice for Parents

Wishes for Baby

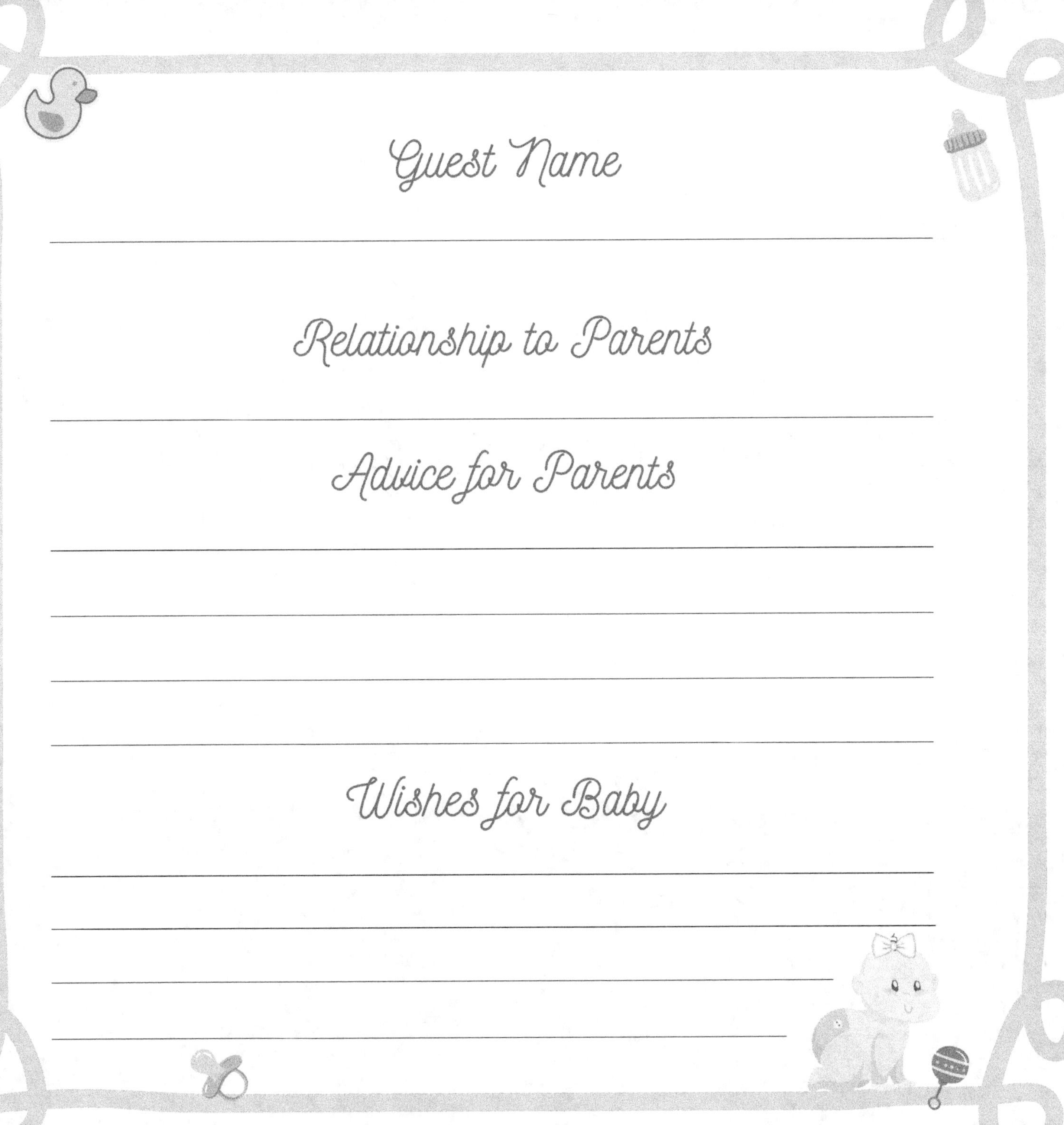

Guest Name
Relationship to Parents
Advice for Parents
Wishes for Baby

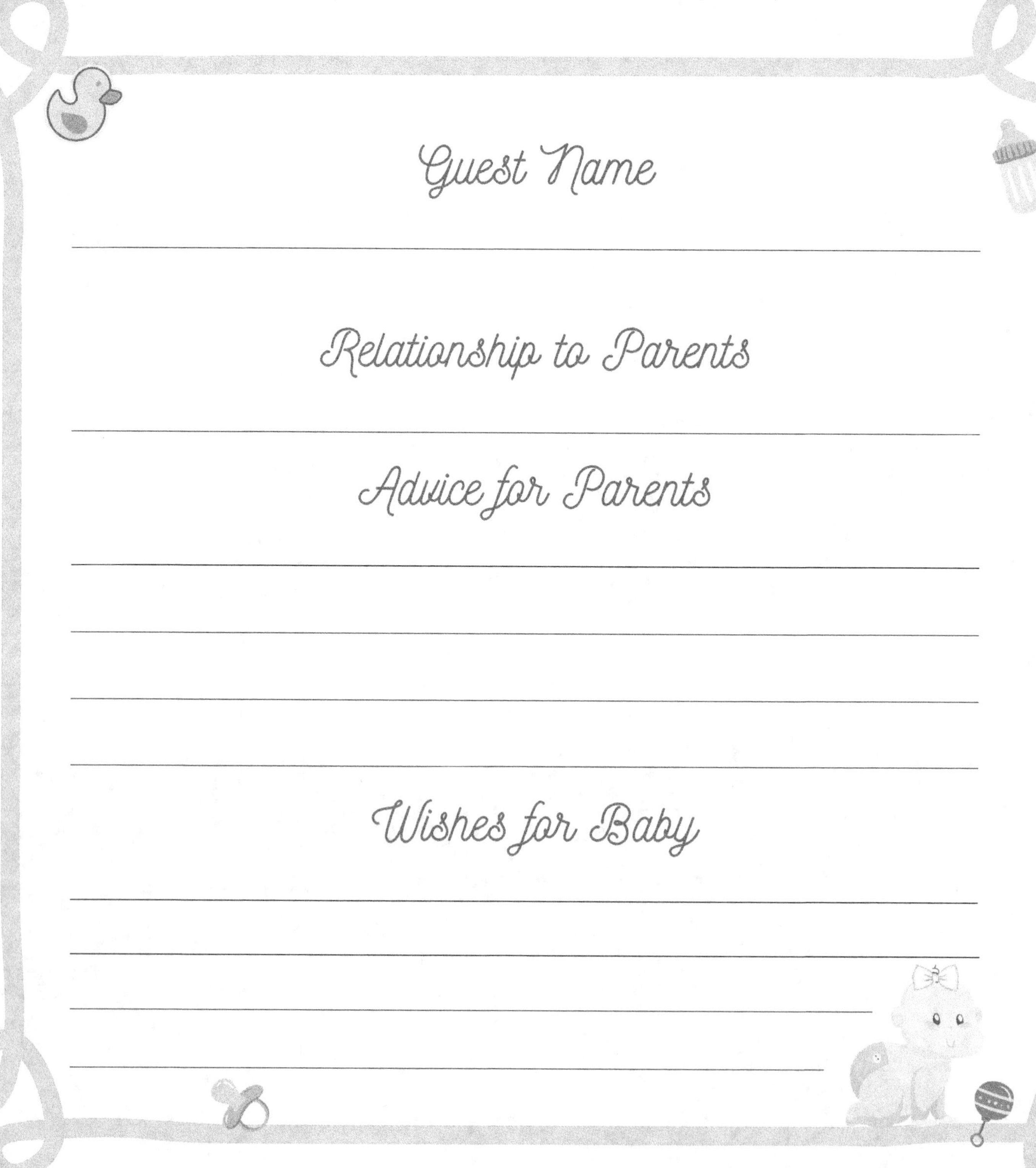

Guest Name
Relationship to Parents
Advice for Parents
Wishes for Baby

Guest Name

Relationship to Parents

Advice for Parents

Wishes for Baby

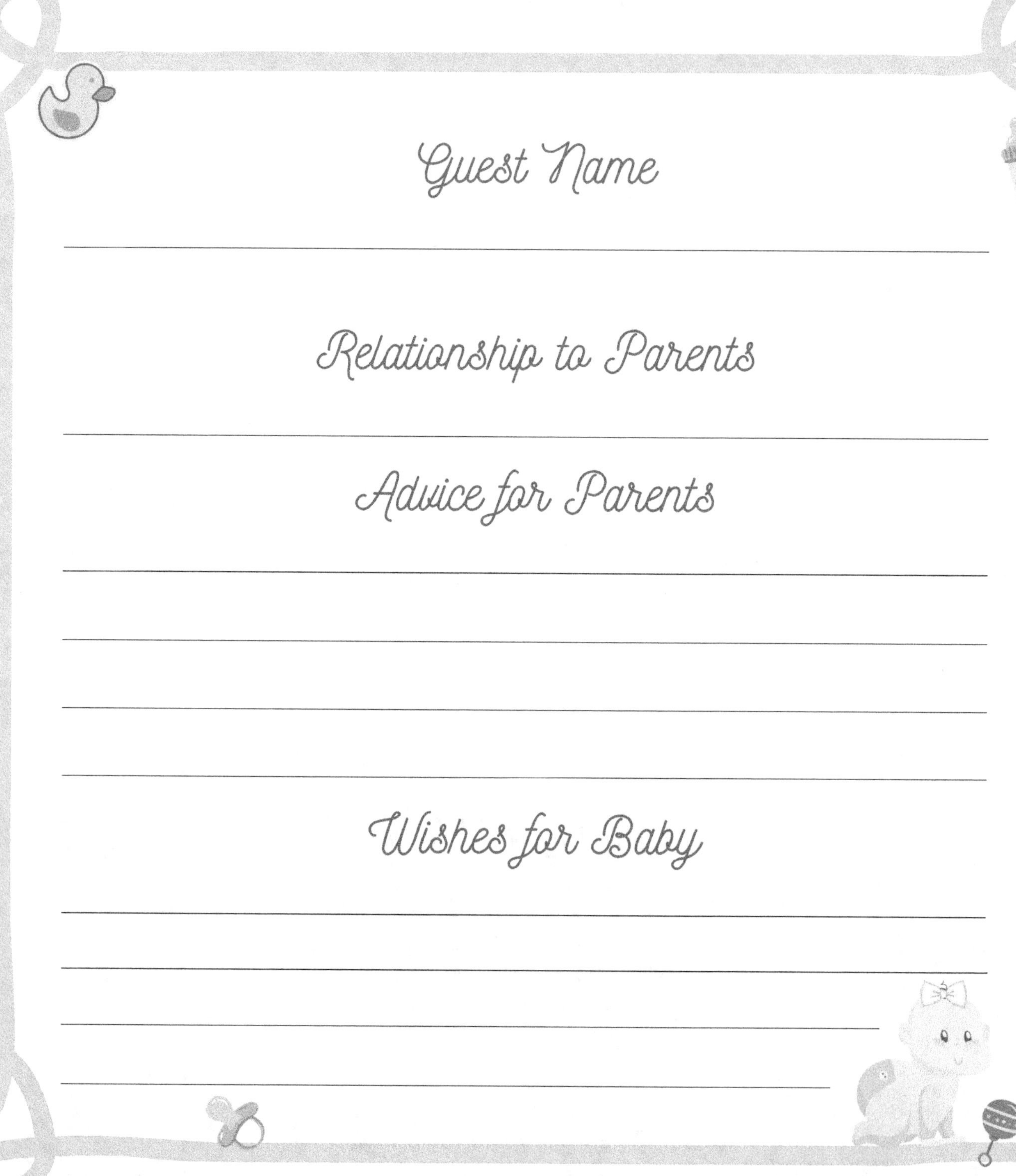

Guest Name

Relationship to Parents

Advice for Parents

Wishes for Baby

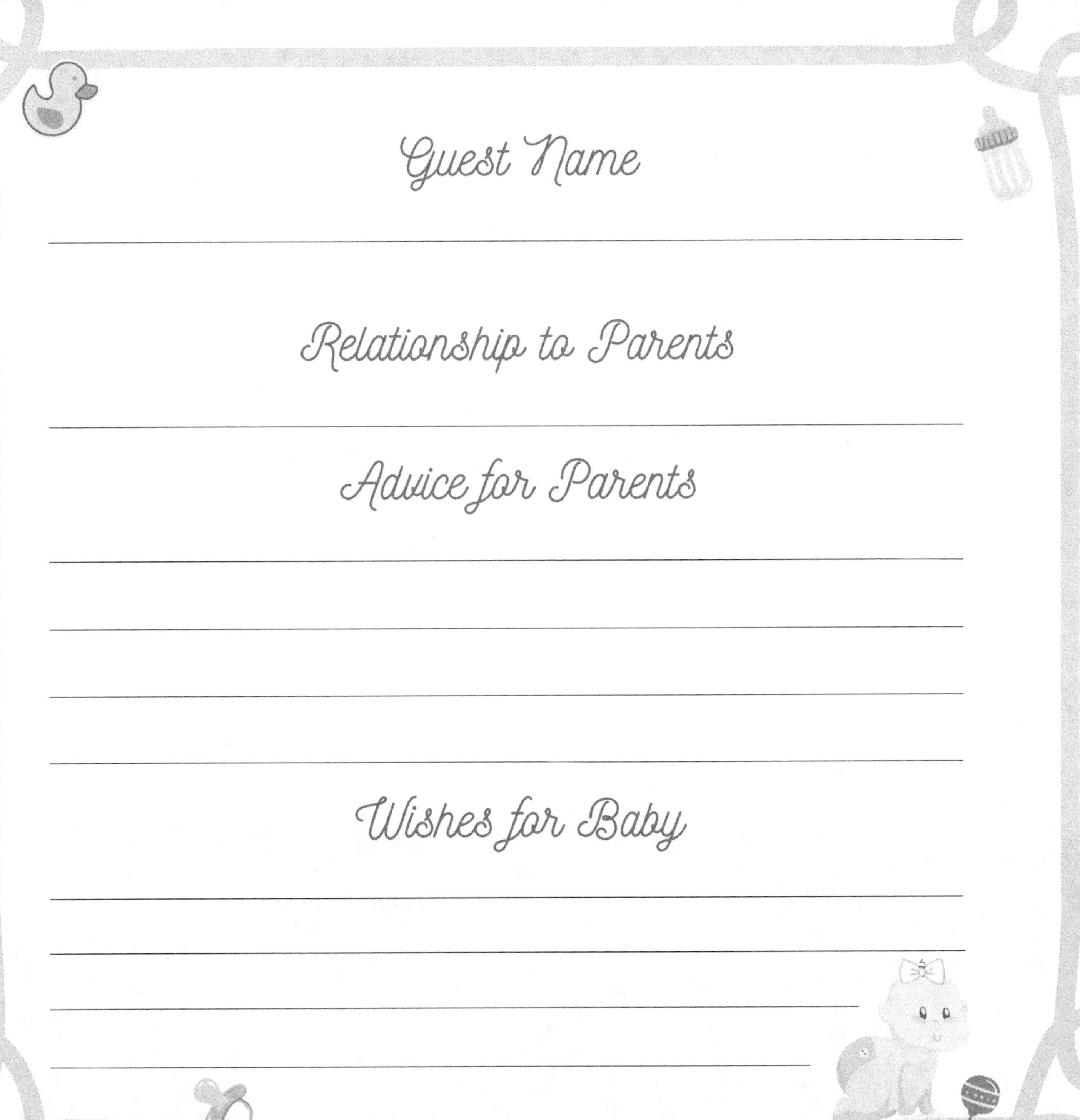

Guest Name
Relationship to Parents
Advice for Parents
Wishes for Baby

Guest Name

Relationship to Parents

Advice for Parents

Wishes for Baby

Guest Name

Relationship to Parents

Advice for Parents

Wishes for Baby

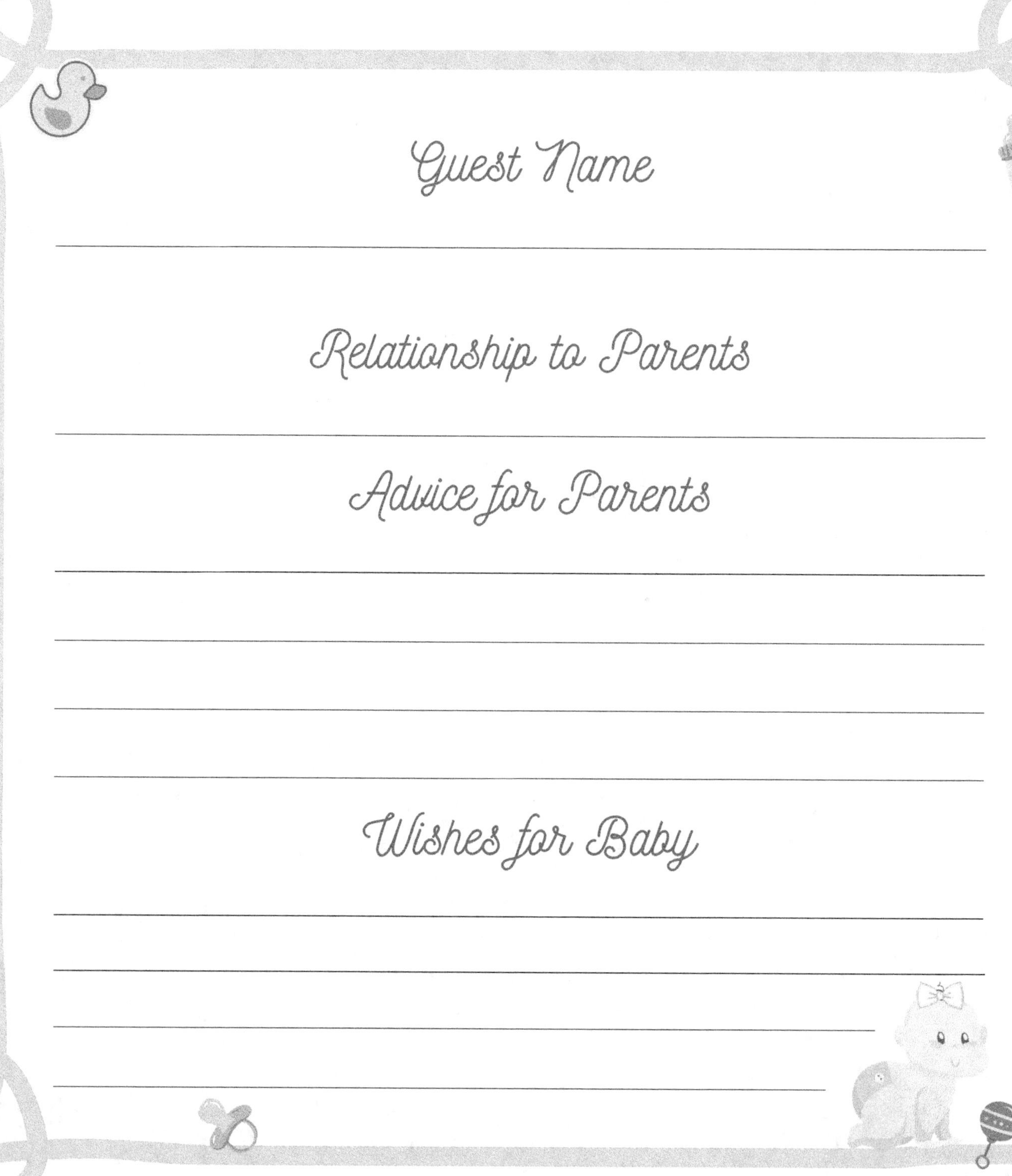

Guest Name

Relationship to Parents

Advice for Parents

Wishes for Baby

Guest Name

____

Relationship to Parents

____

Advice for Parents

____

____

____

Wishes for Baby

____

____

____

Guest Name

Relationship to Parents

Advice for Parents

Wishes for Baby

Guest Name

____

Relationship to Parents

____

Advice for Parents

____

____

____

Wishes for Baby

____

____

____

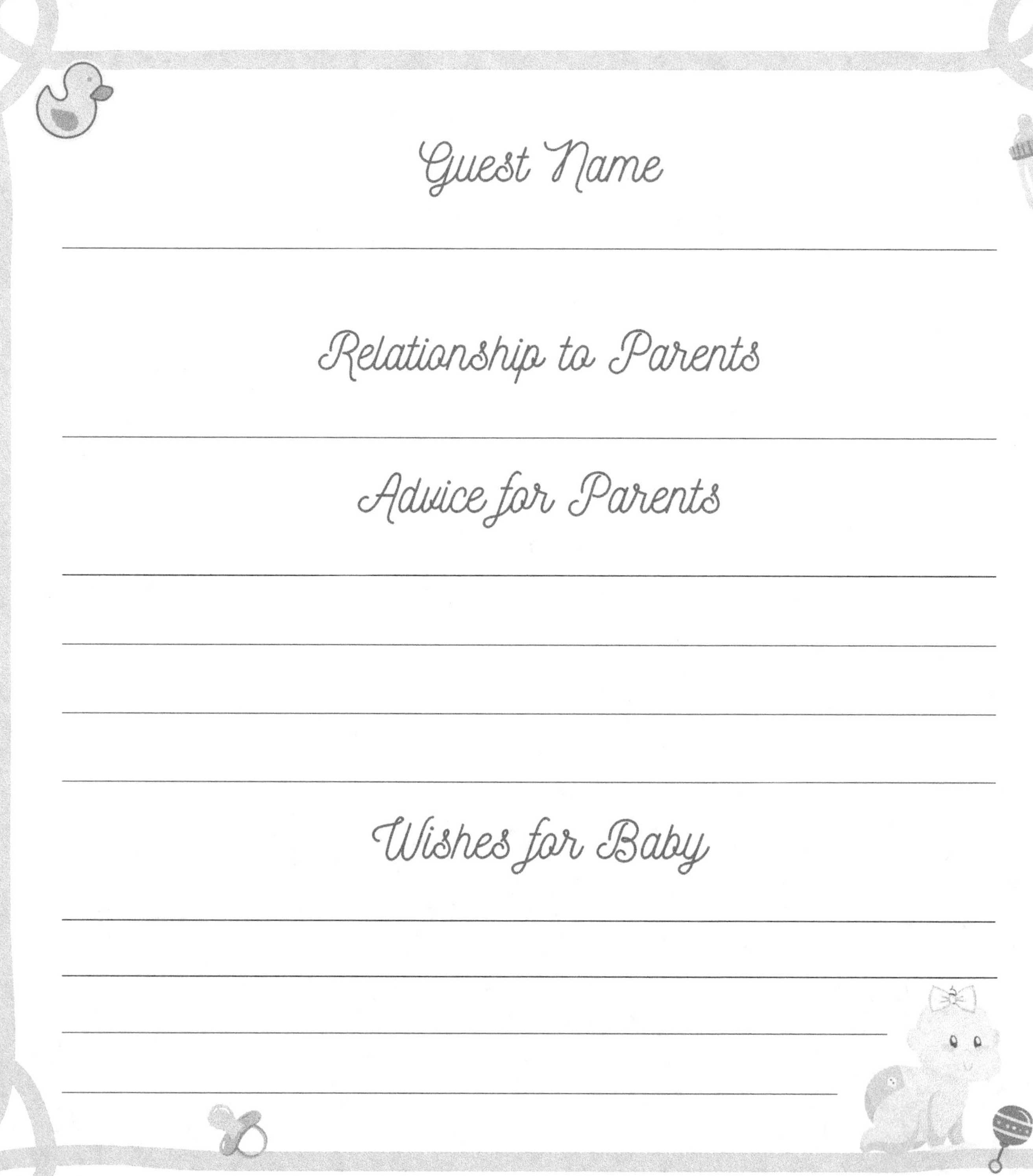

Guest Name
Relationship to Parents
Advice for Parents
Wishes for Baby

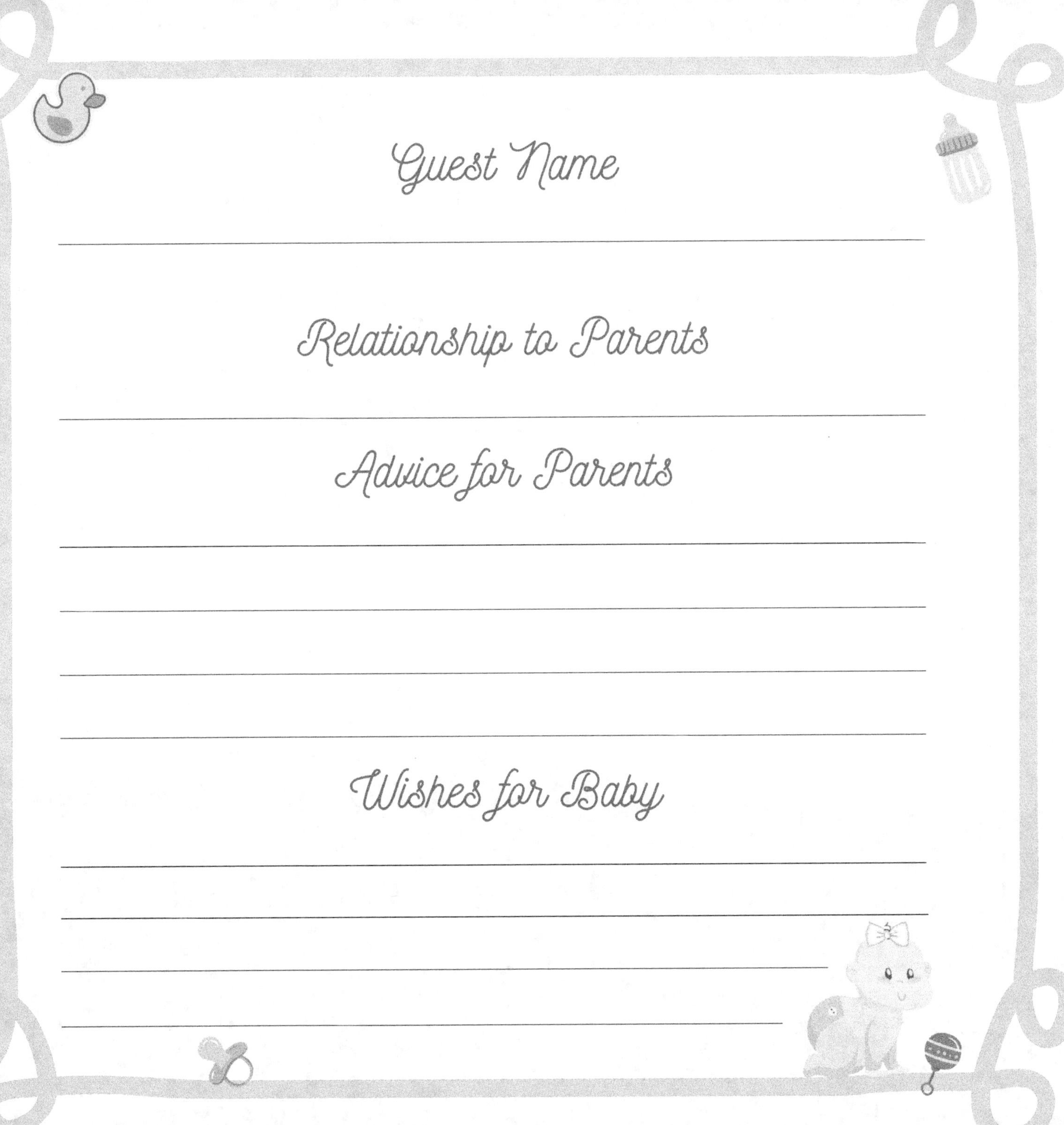
Guest Name
Relationship to Parents
Advice for Parents
Wishes for Baby

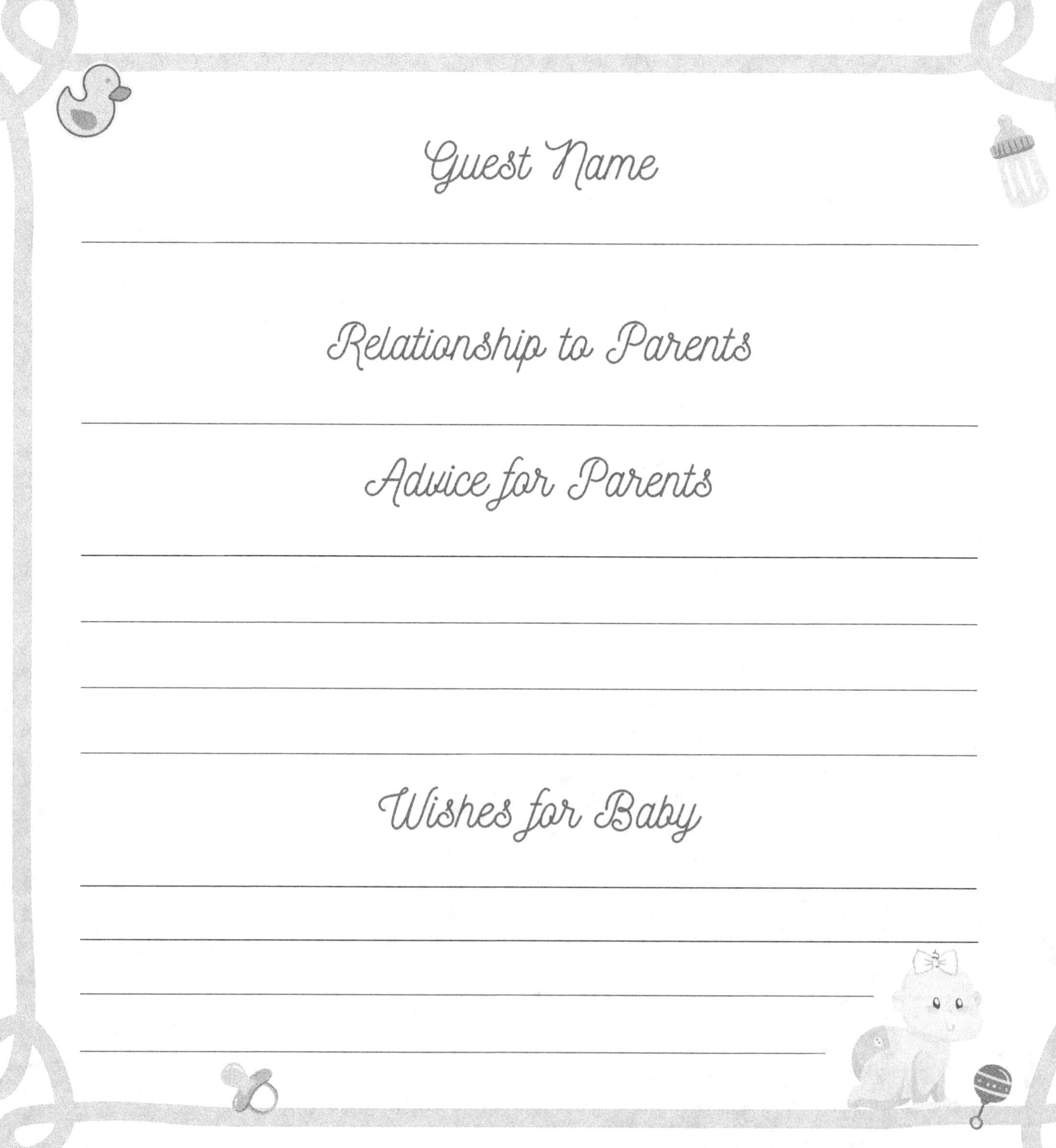

Guest Name
Relationship to Parents
Advice for Parents
Wishes for Baby

Guest Name

Relationship to Parents

Advice for Parents

Wishes for Baby

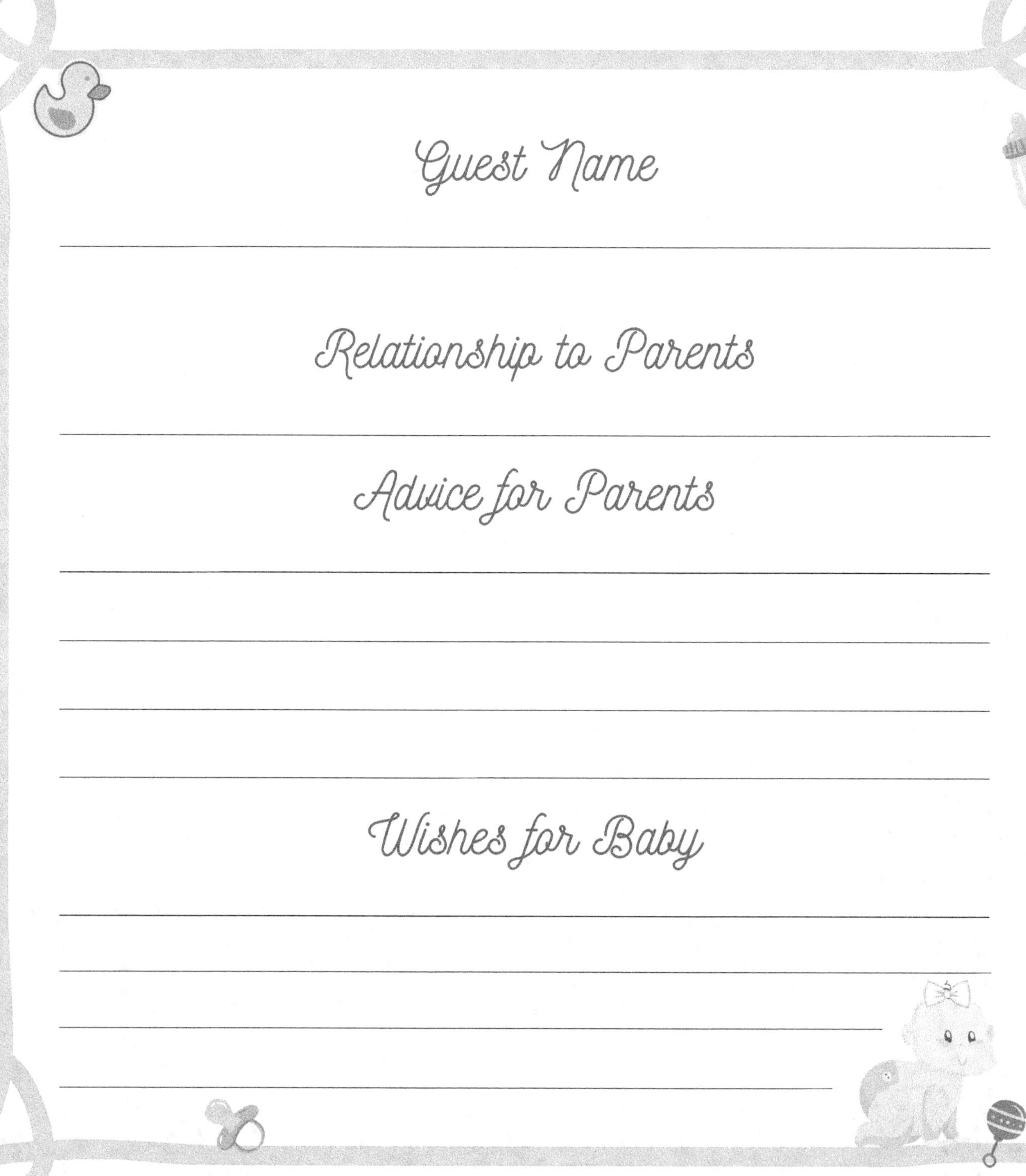

Guest Name

Relationship to Parents

Advice for Parents

Wishes for Baby

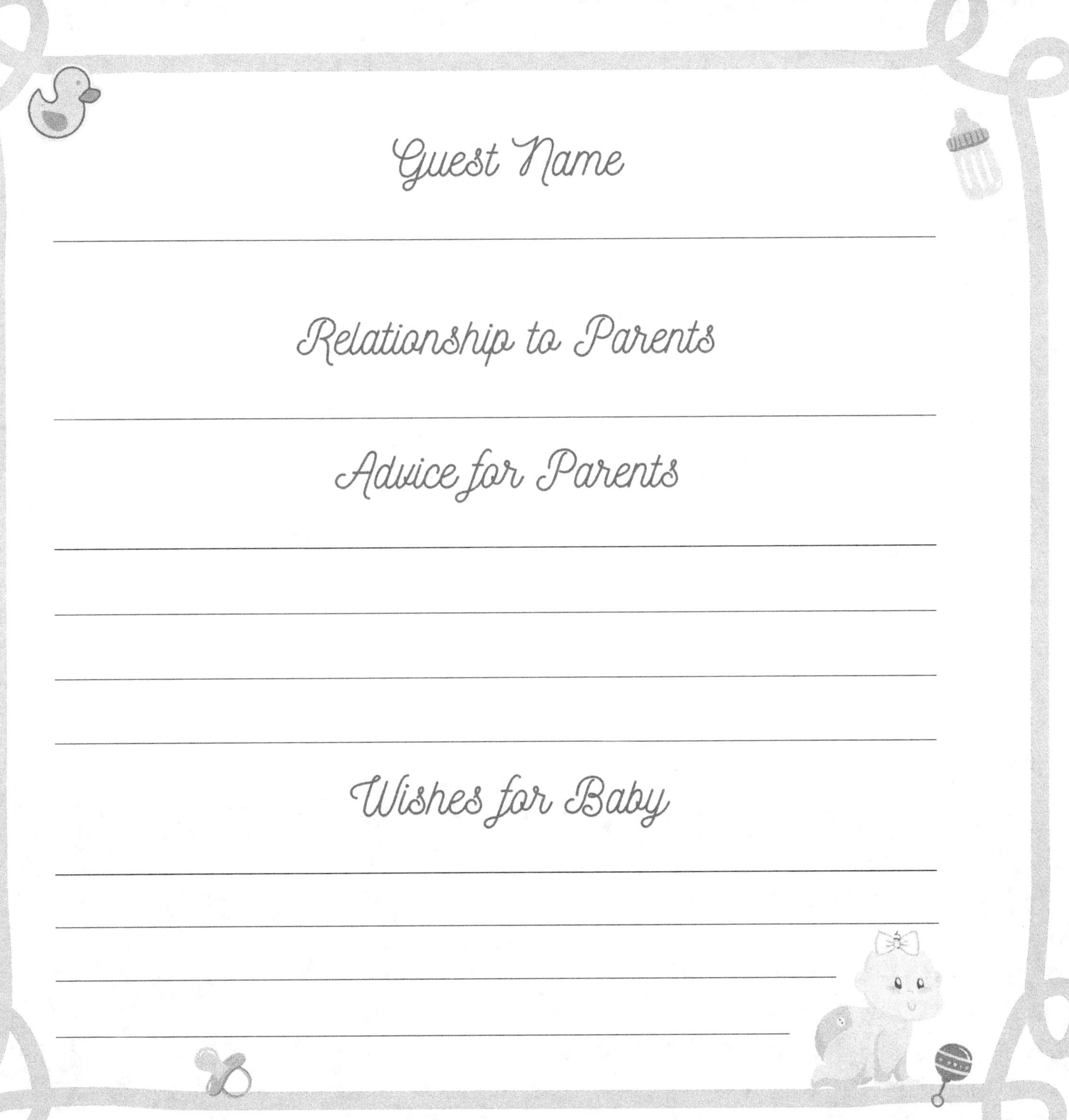

Guest Name

Relationship to Parents

Advice for Parents

Wishes for Baby

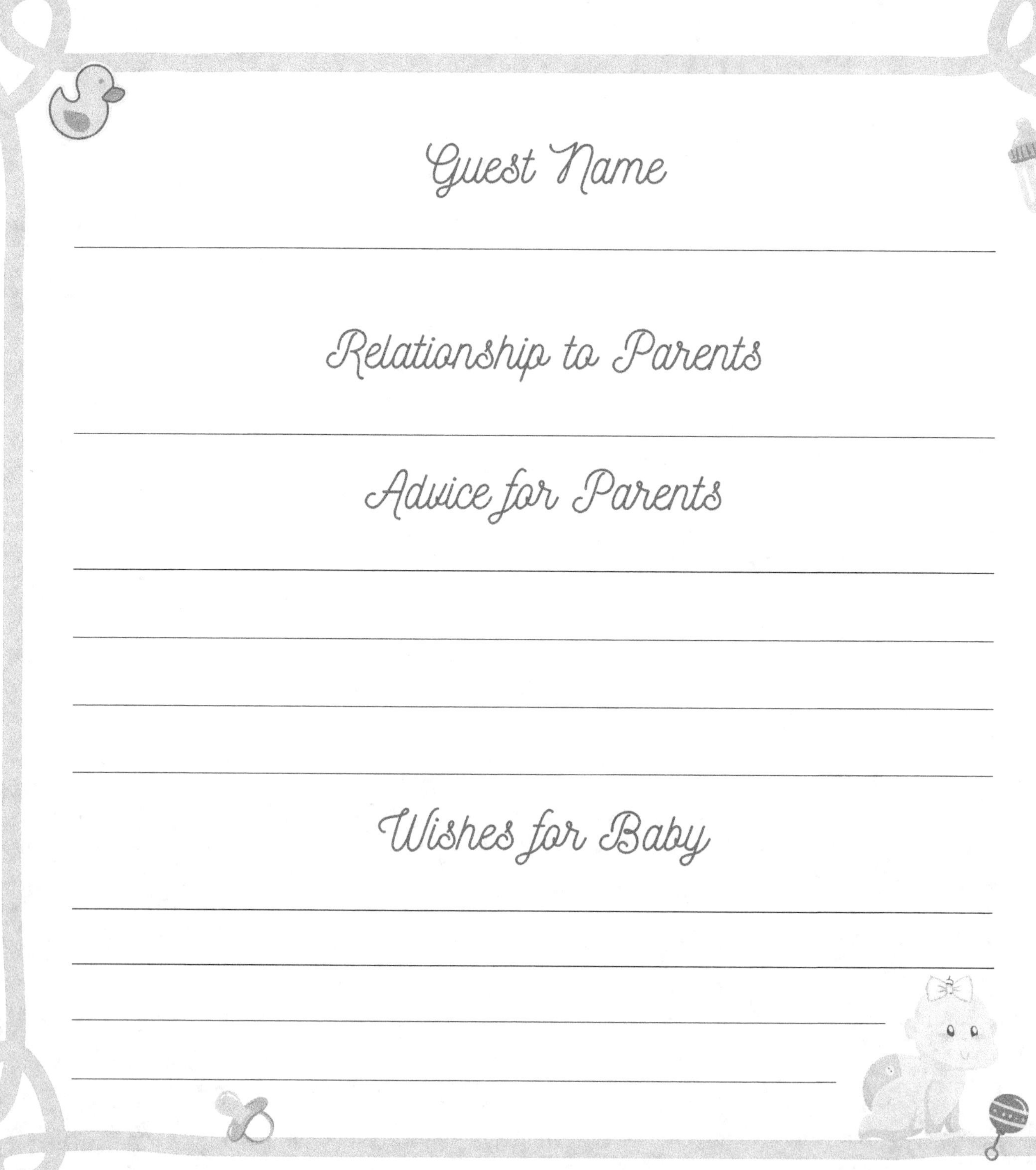
Guest Name

Relationship to Parents

Advice for Parents

Wishes for Baby

Guest Name

Relationship to Parents

Advice for Parents

Wishes for Baby

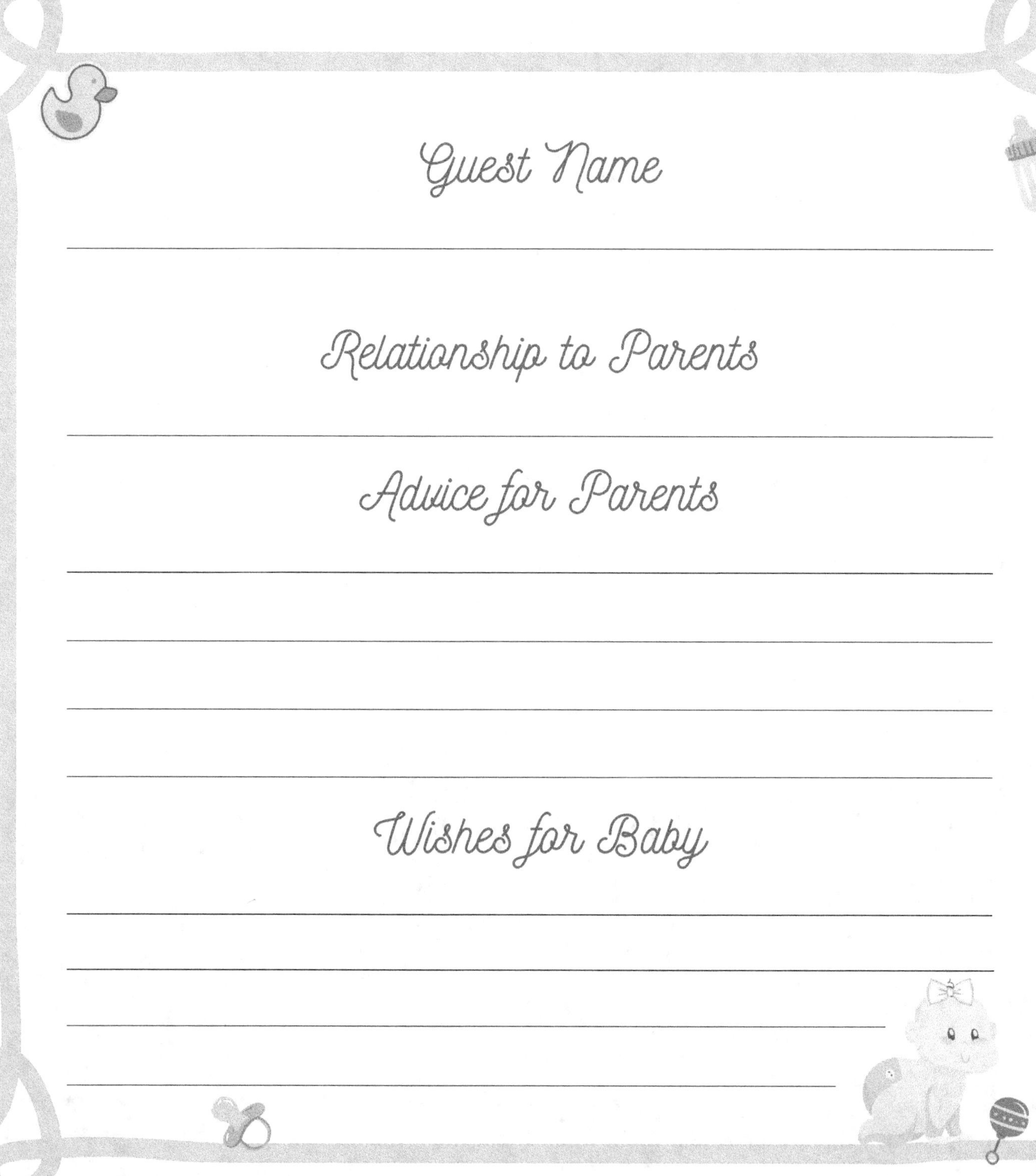

Guest Name

Relationship to Parents

Advice for Parents

Wishes for Baby

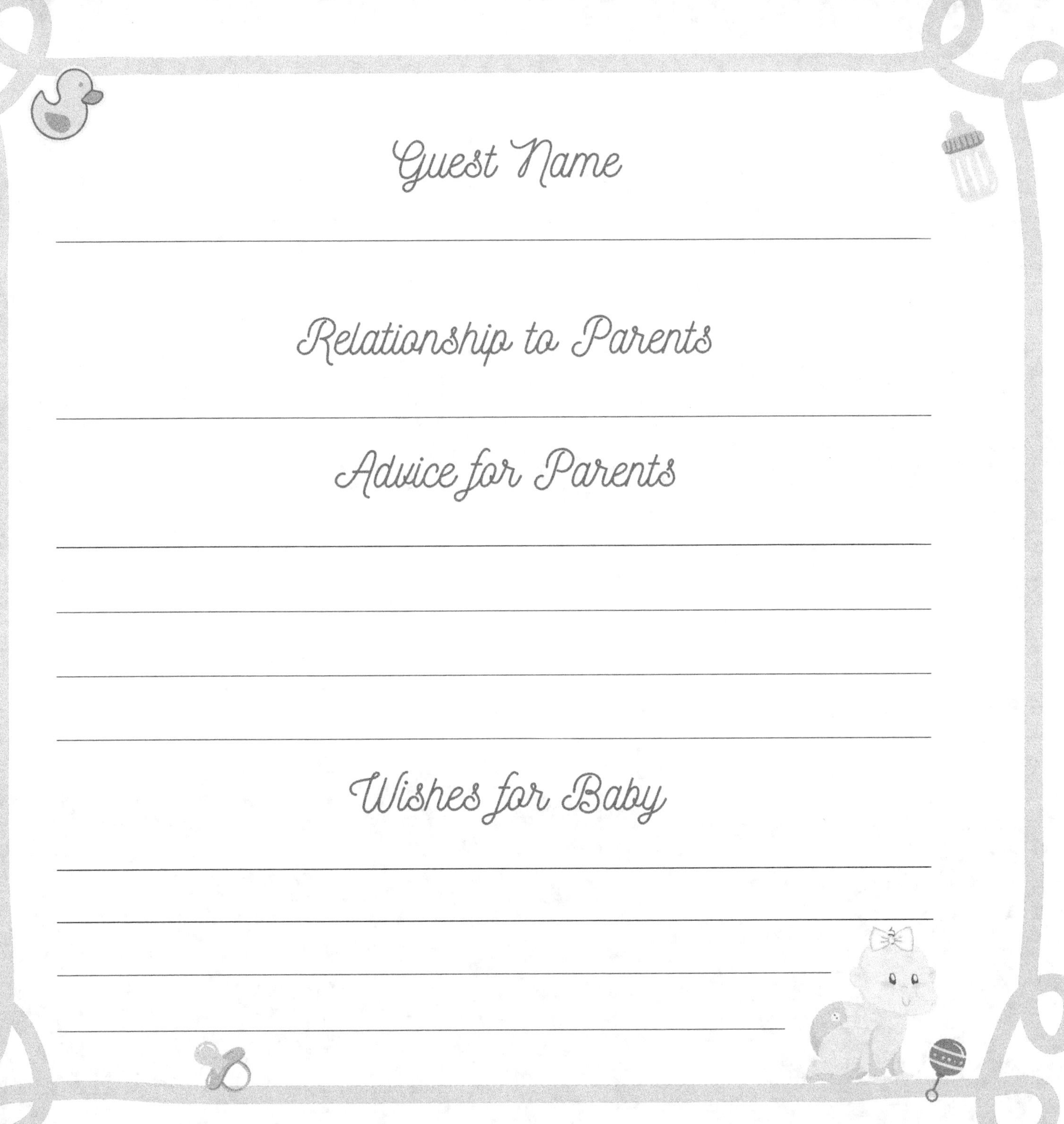

Guest Name
Relationship to Parents
Advice for Parents
Wishes for Baby

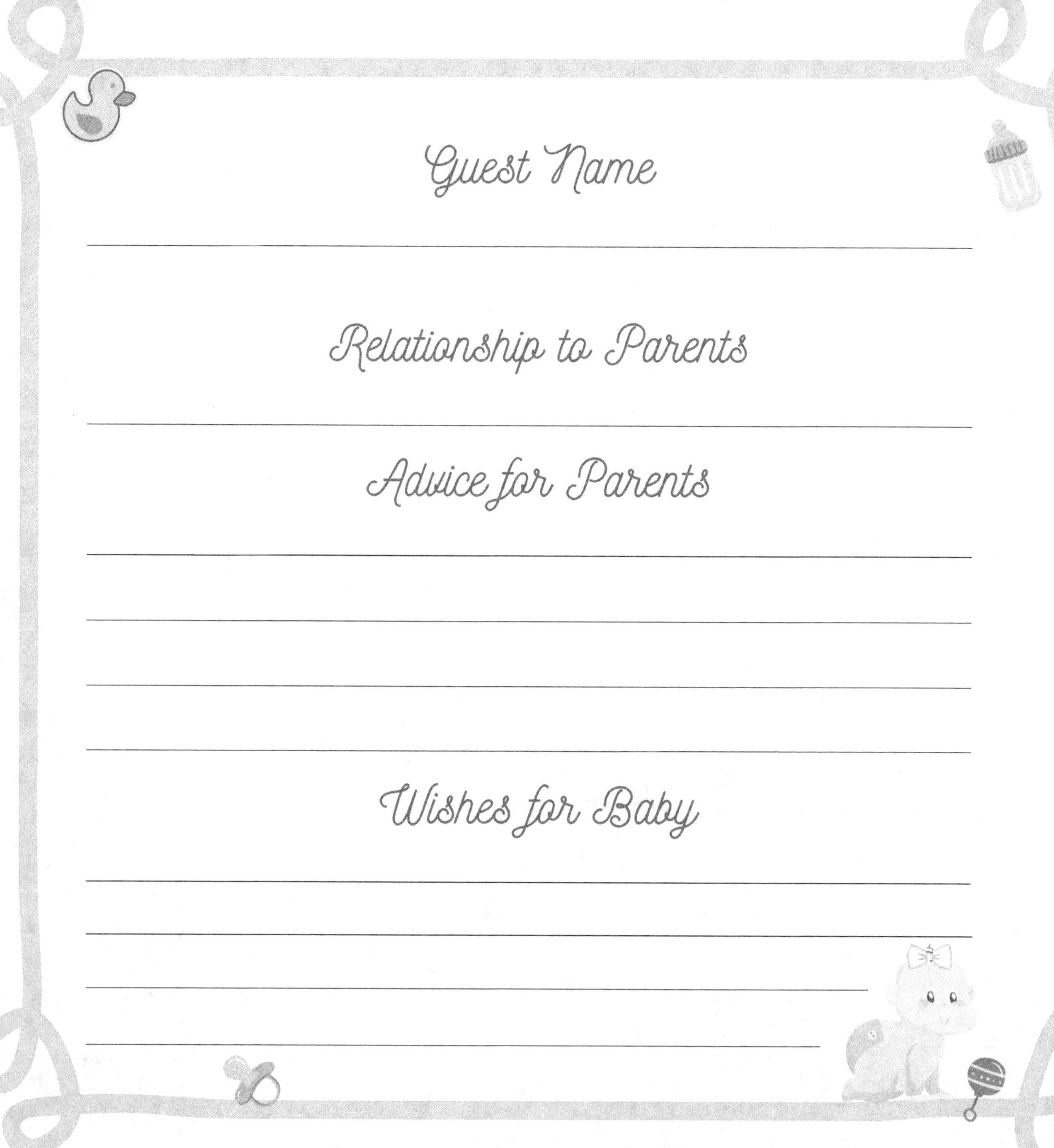
Guest Name

Relationship to Parents

Advice for Parents

Wishes for Baby

Guest Name

____

Relationship to Parents

____

Advice for Parents

____

____

____

Wishes for Baby

____

____

____

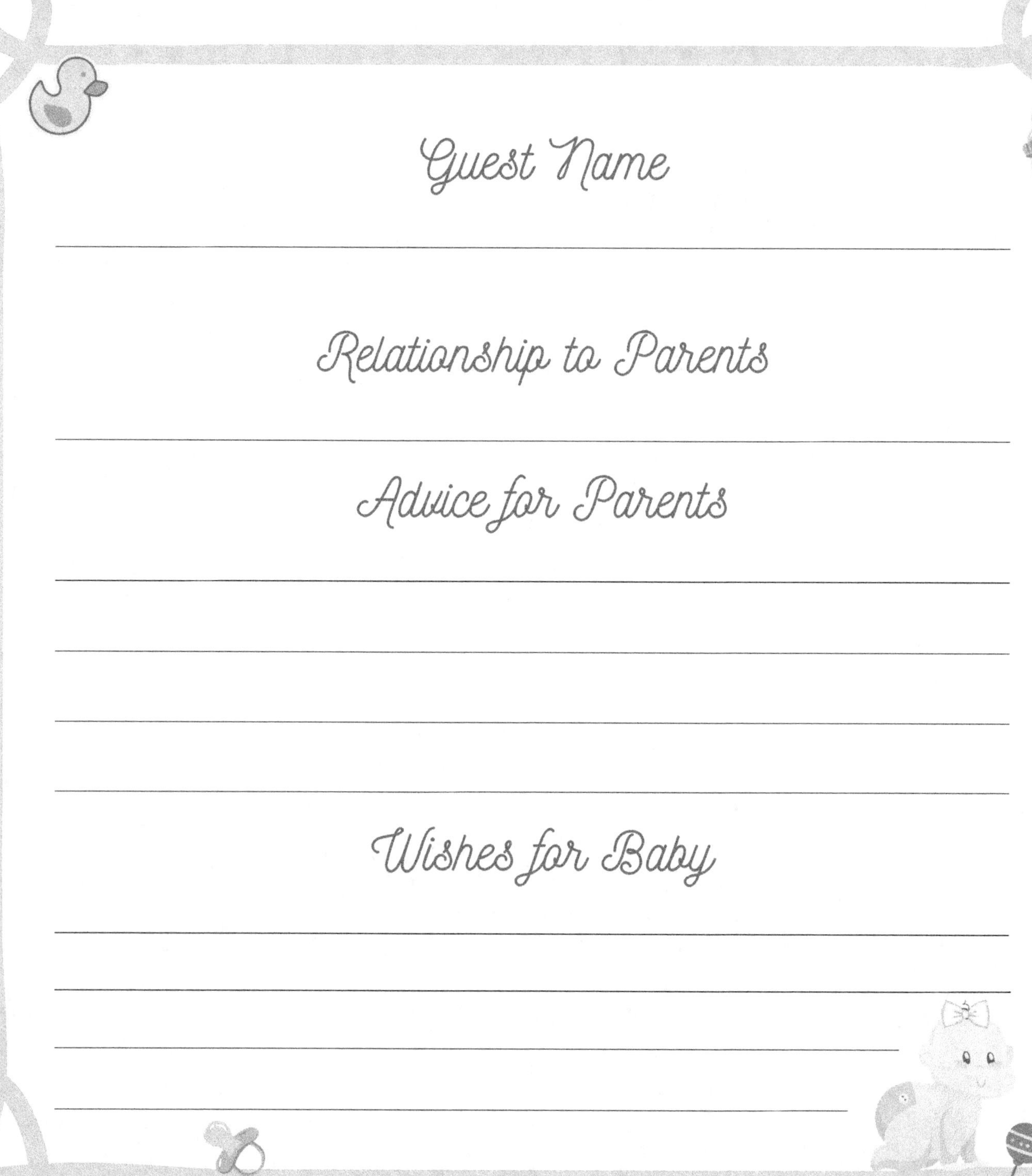
Guest Name

Relationship to Parents

Advice for Parents

Wishes for Baby

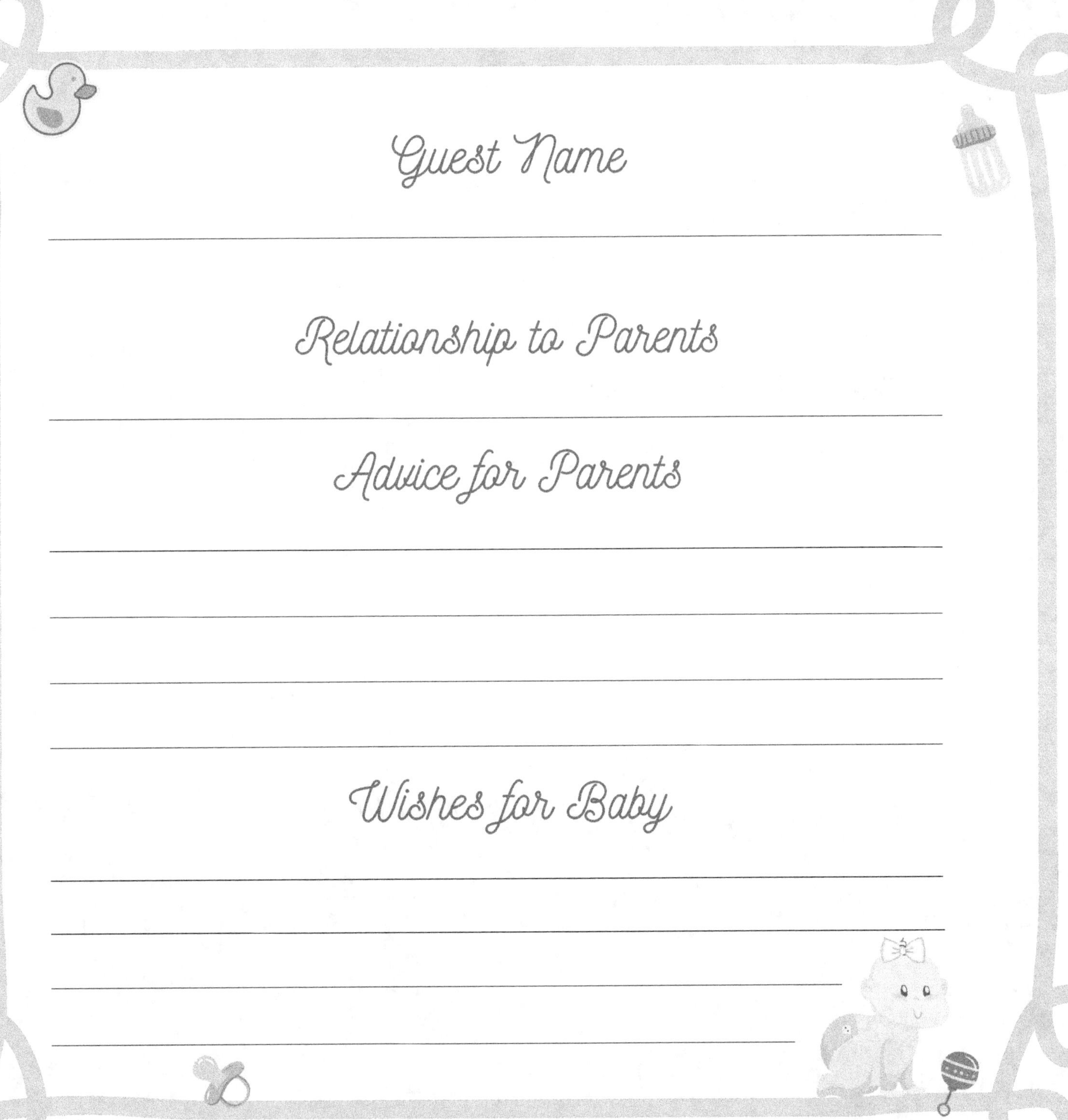Guest Name

Relationship to Parents

Advice for Parents

Wishes for Baby

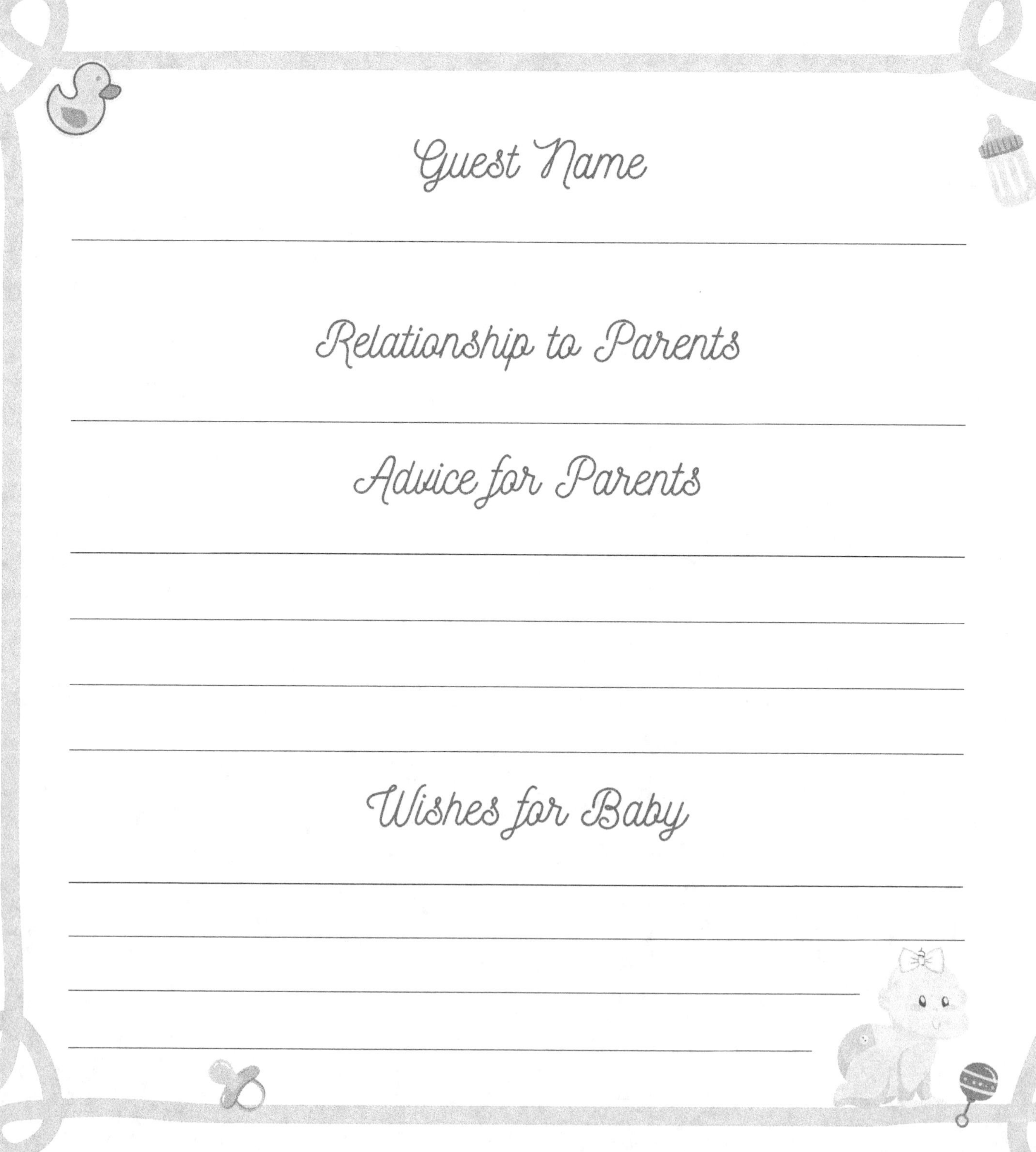
Guest Name

Relationship to Parents

Advice for Parents

Wishes for Baby

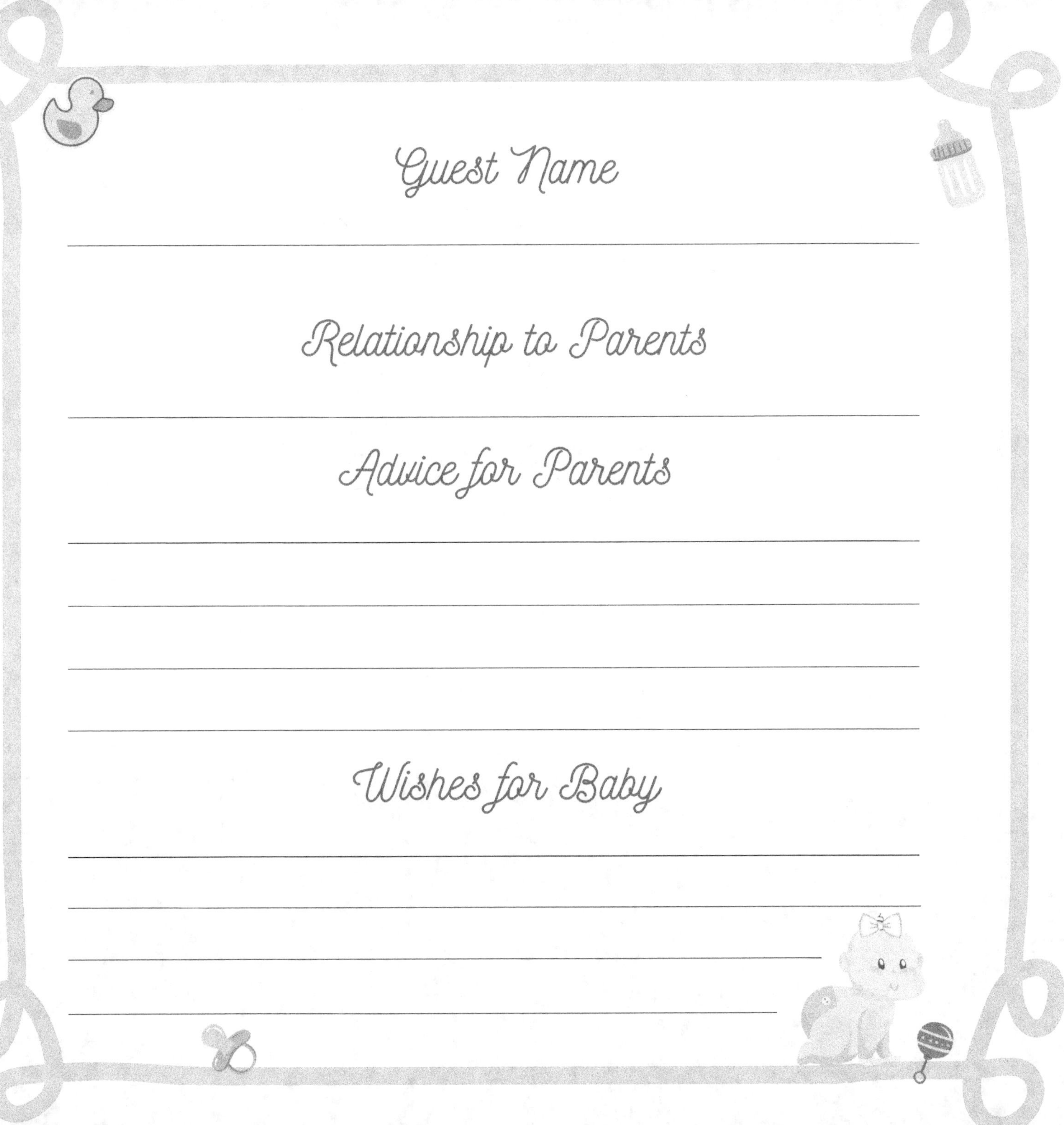
Guest Name
Relationship to Parents
Advice for Parents
Wishes for Baby

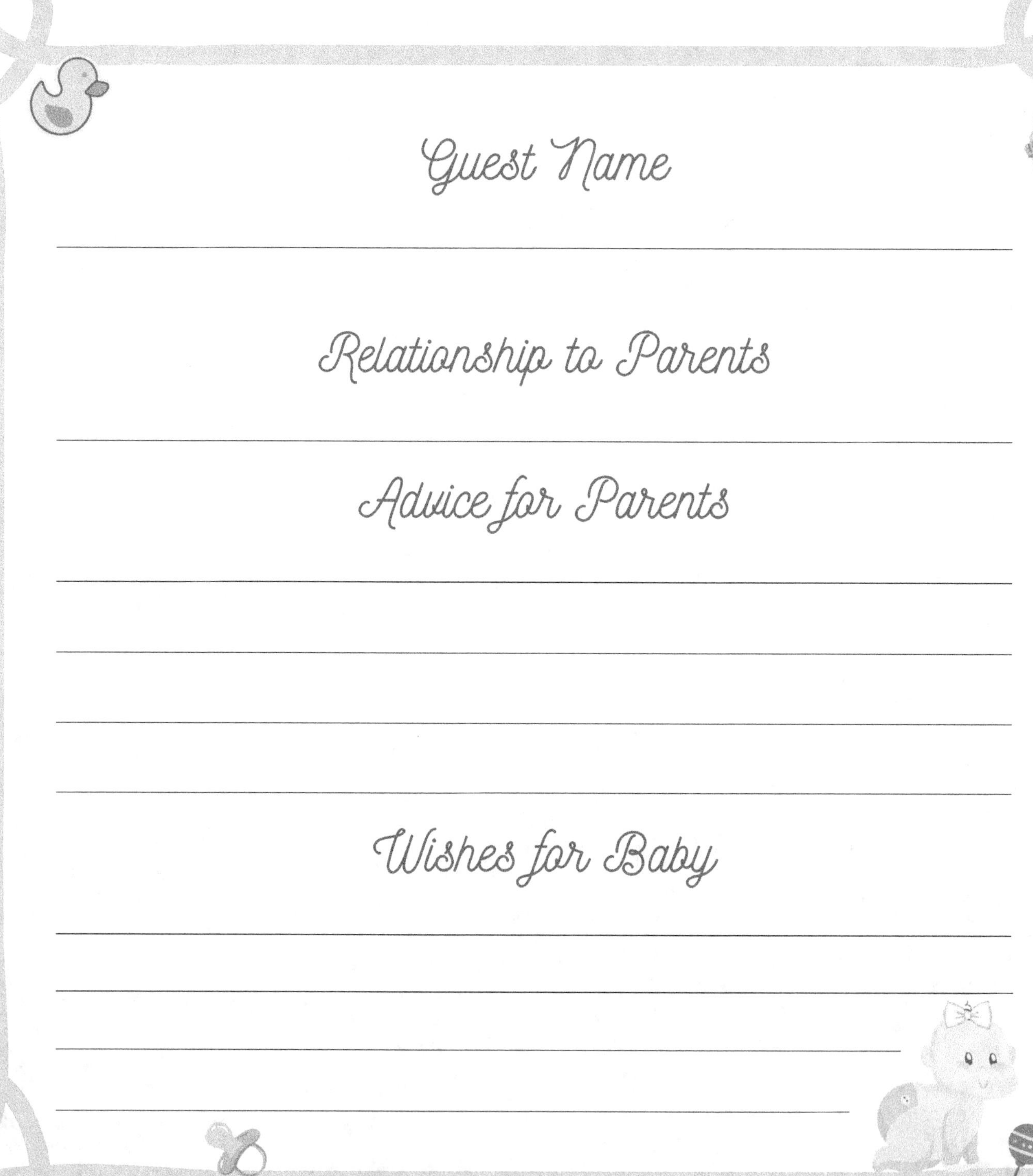

Guest Name

Relationship to Parents

Advice for Parents

Wishes for Baby

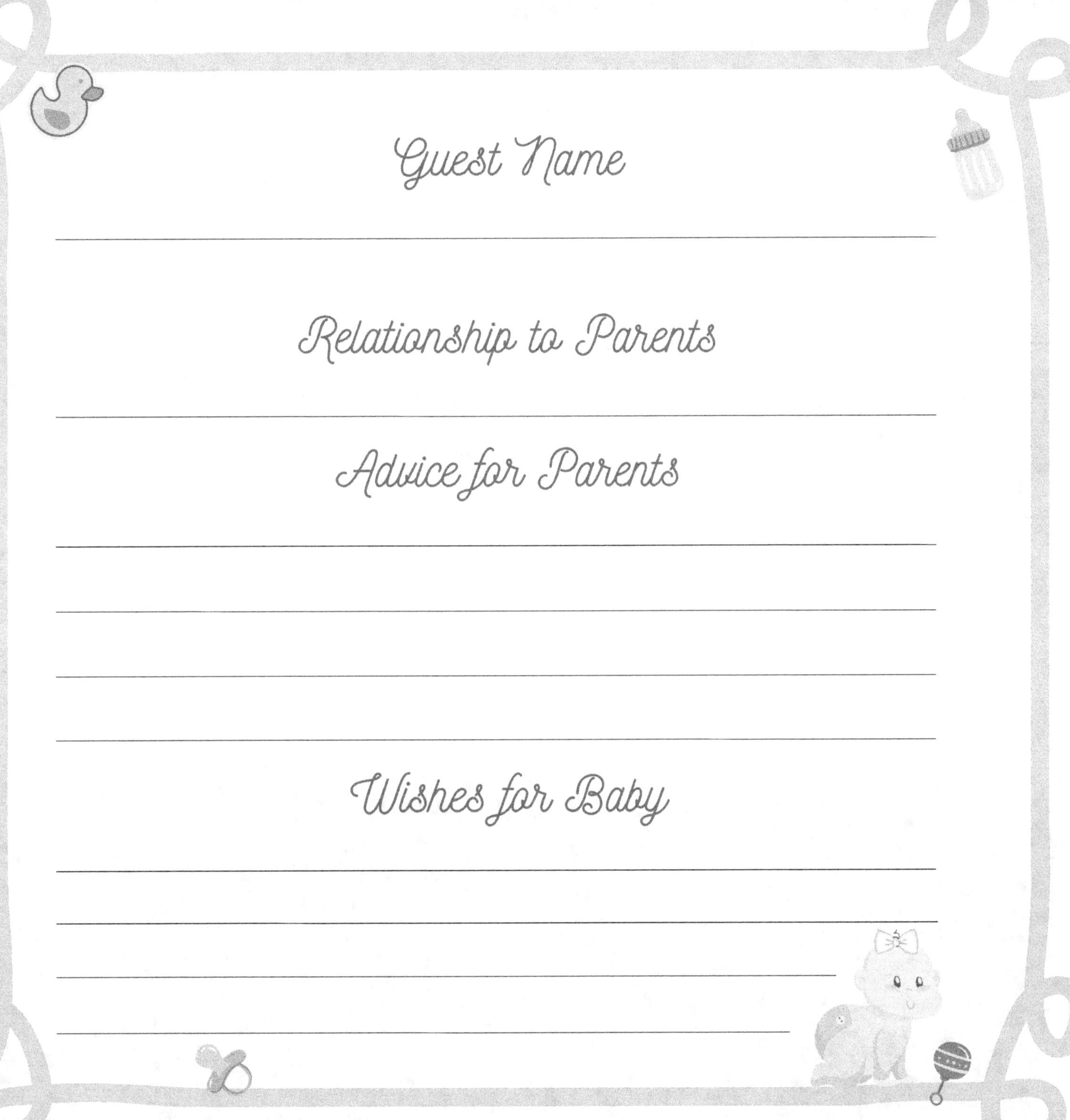

Guest Name
Relationship to Parents
Advice for Parents
Wishes for Baby

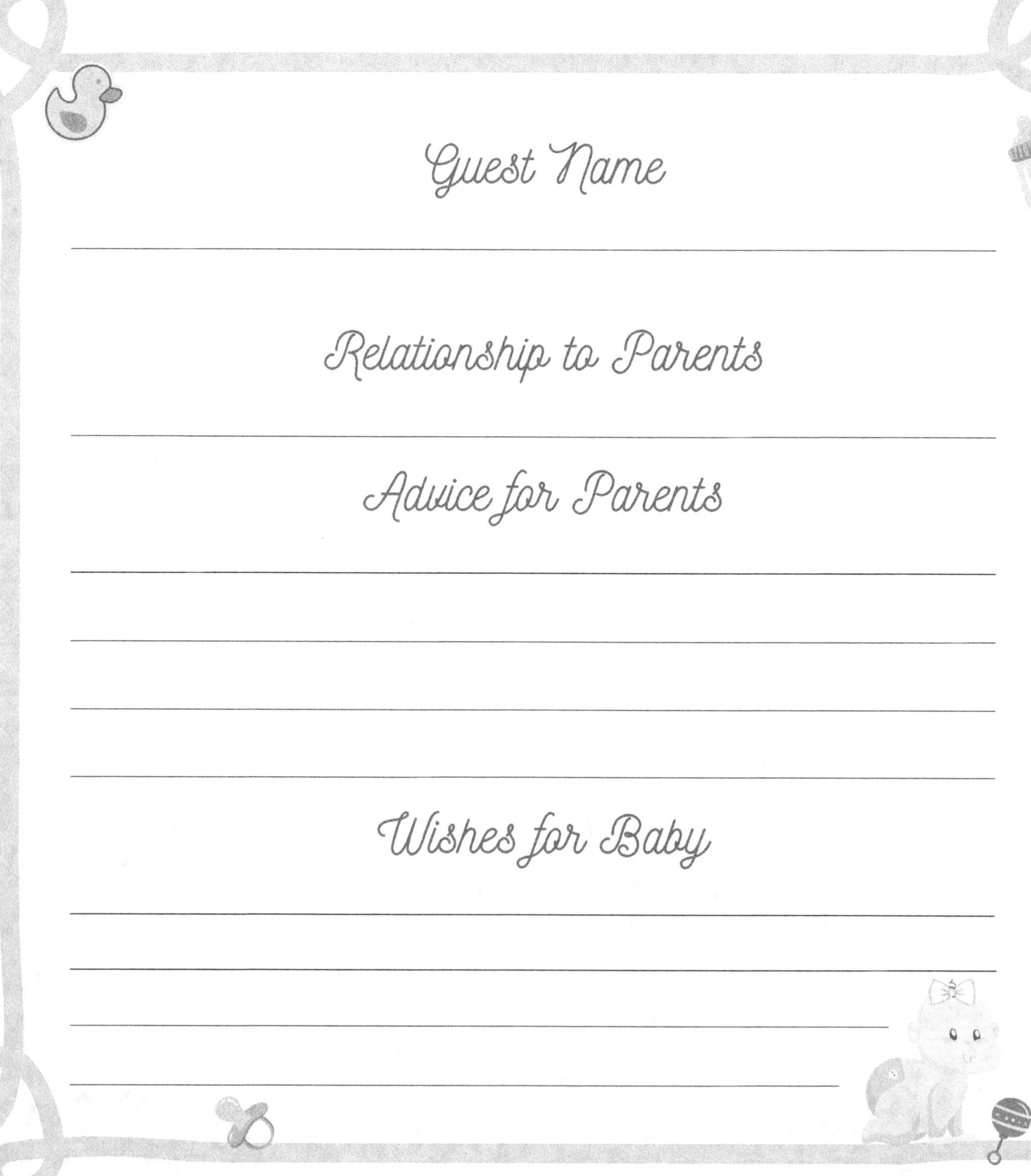

Guest Name

Relationship to Parents

Advice for Parents

Wishes for Baby

Guest Name

Relationship to Parents

Advice for Parents

Wishes for Baby

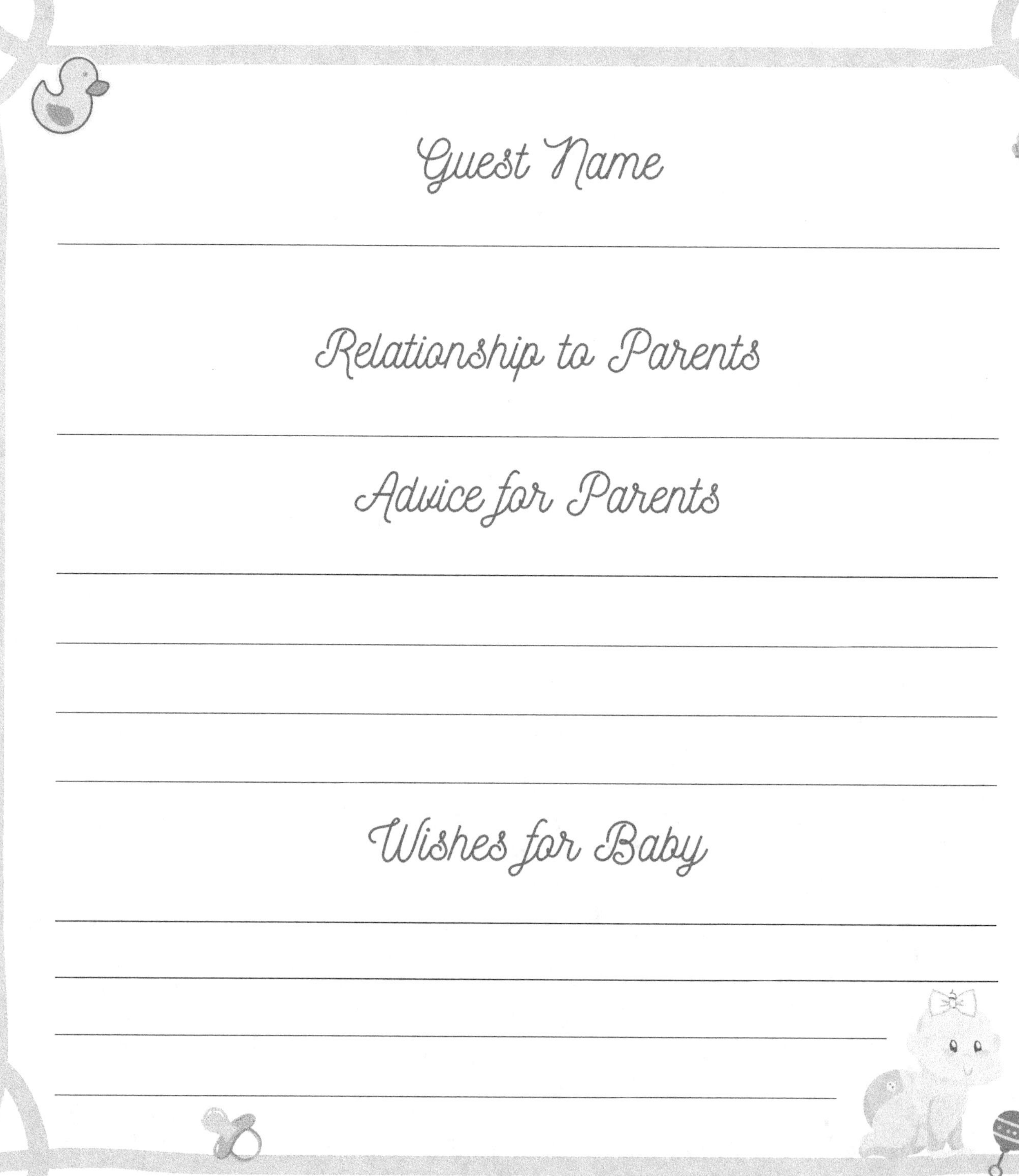

Guest Name

Relationship to Parents

Advice for Parents

Wishes for Baby

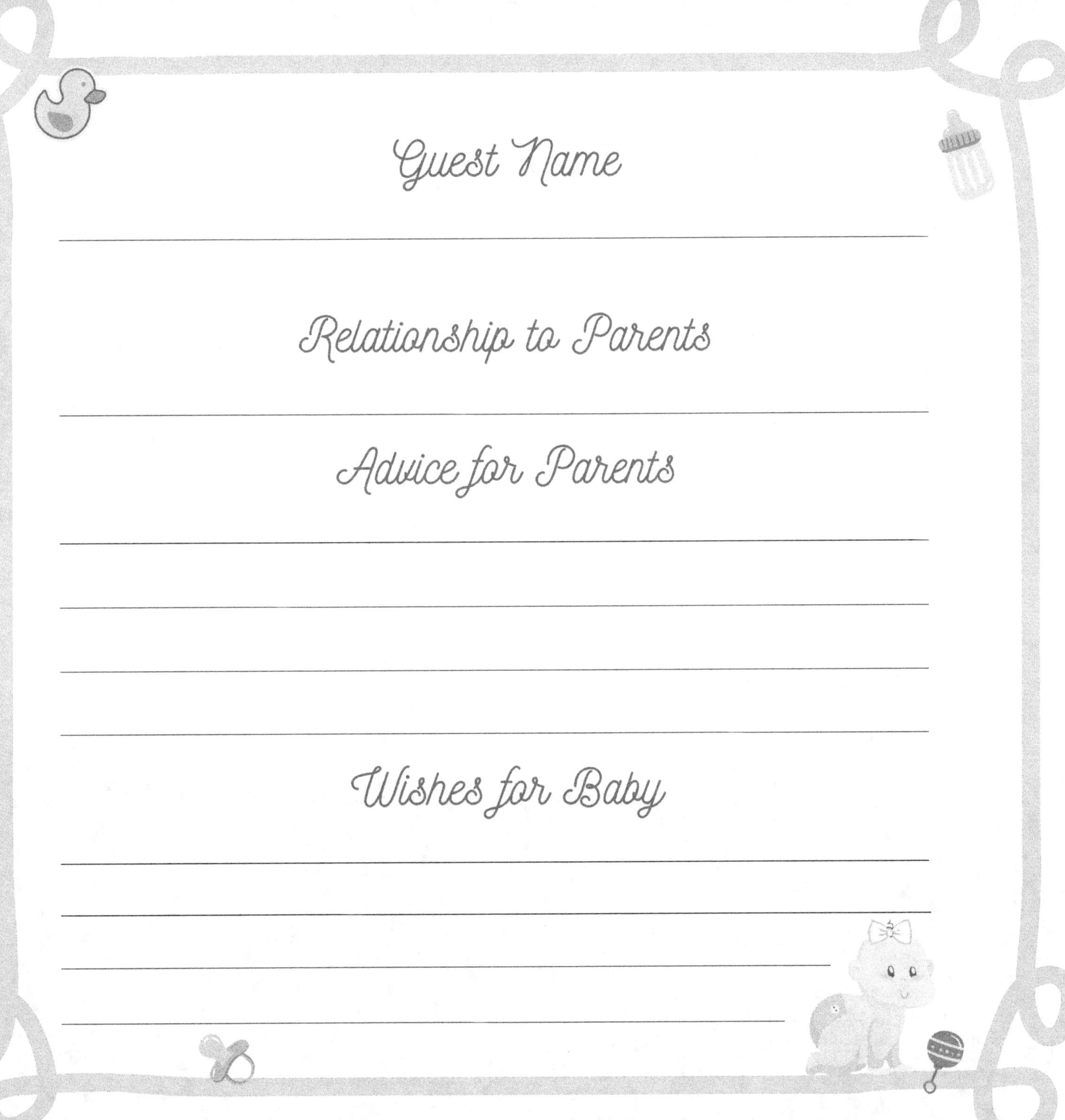

Guest Name

Relationship to Parents

Advice for Parents

Wishes for Baby

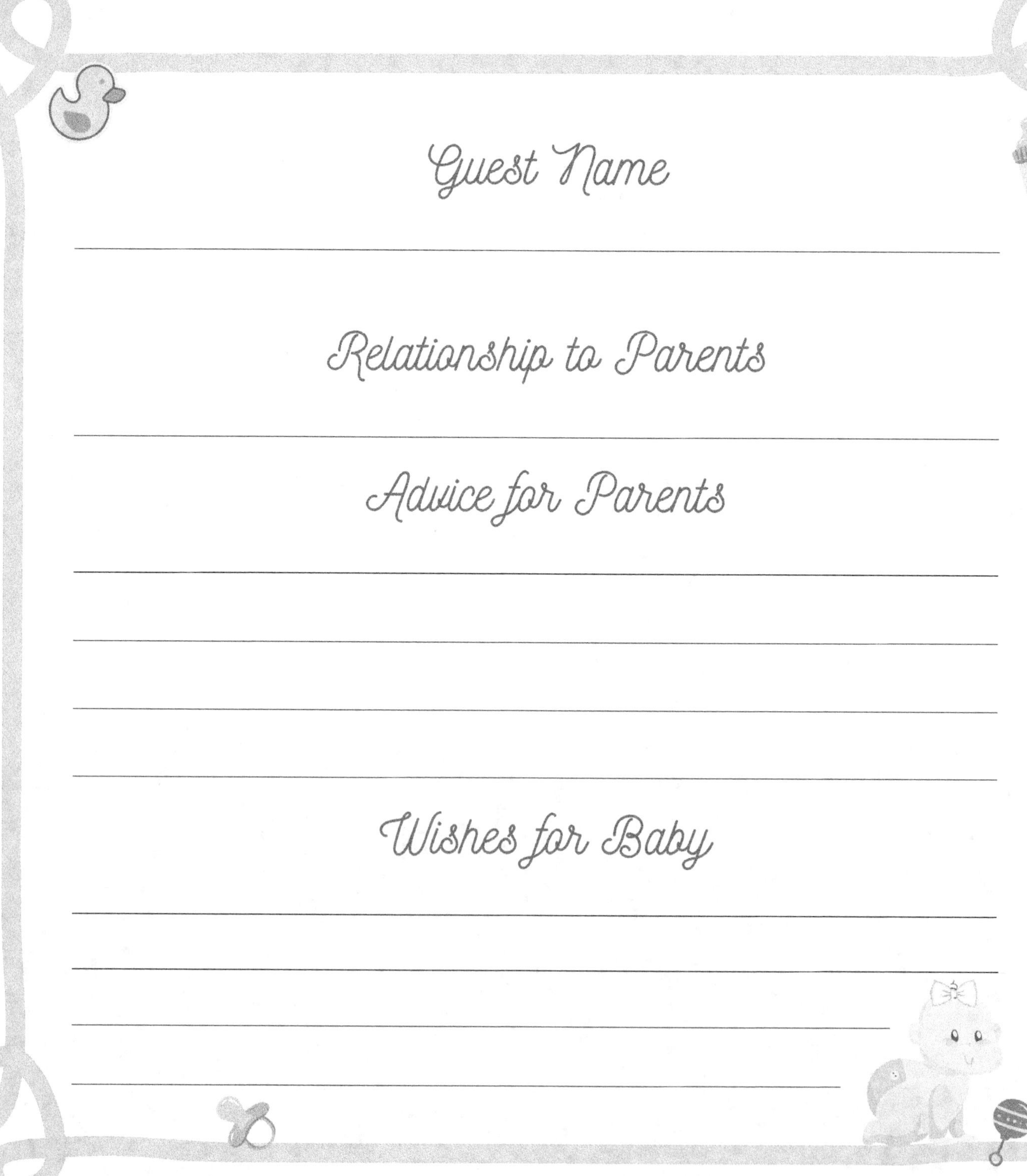

Guest Name
Relationship to Parents
Advice for Parents
Wishes for Baby

Guest Name

Relationship to Parents

Advice for Parents

Wishes for Baby

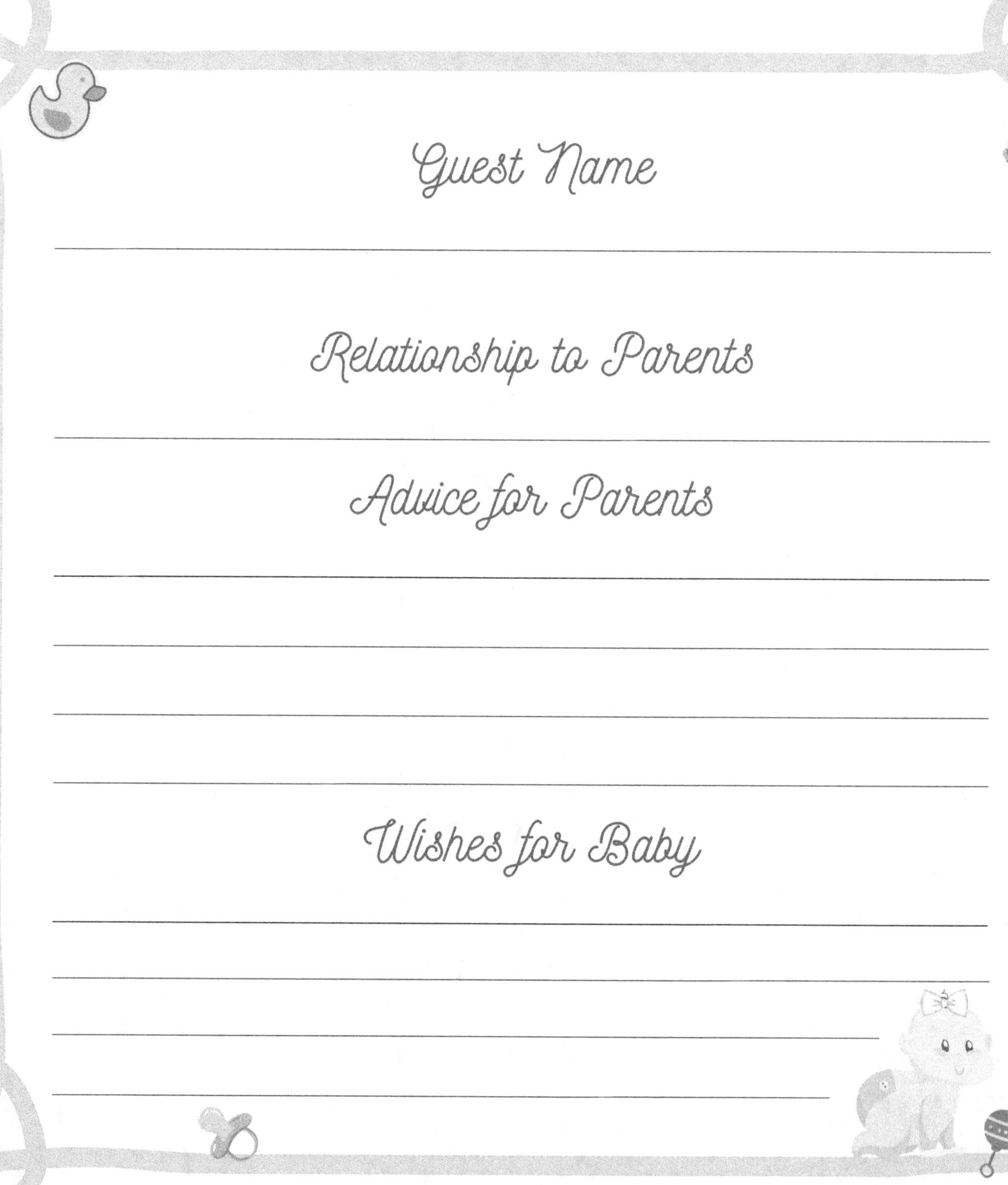

Guest Name

Relationship to Parents

Advice for Parents

Wishes for Baby

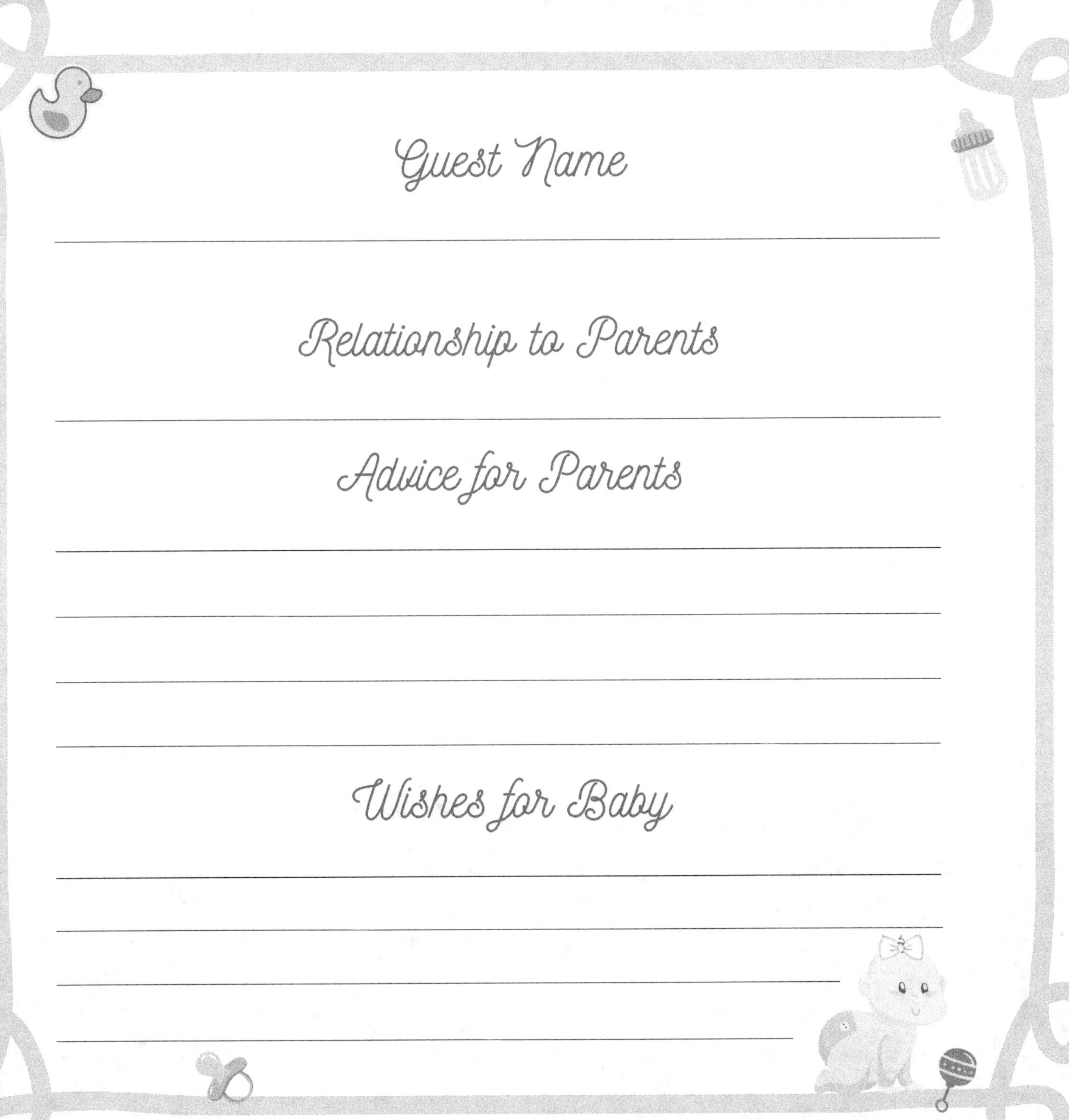

Guest Name
Relationship to Parents
Advice for Parents
Wishes for Baby

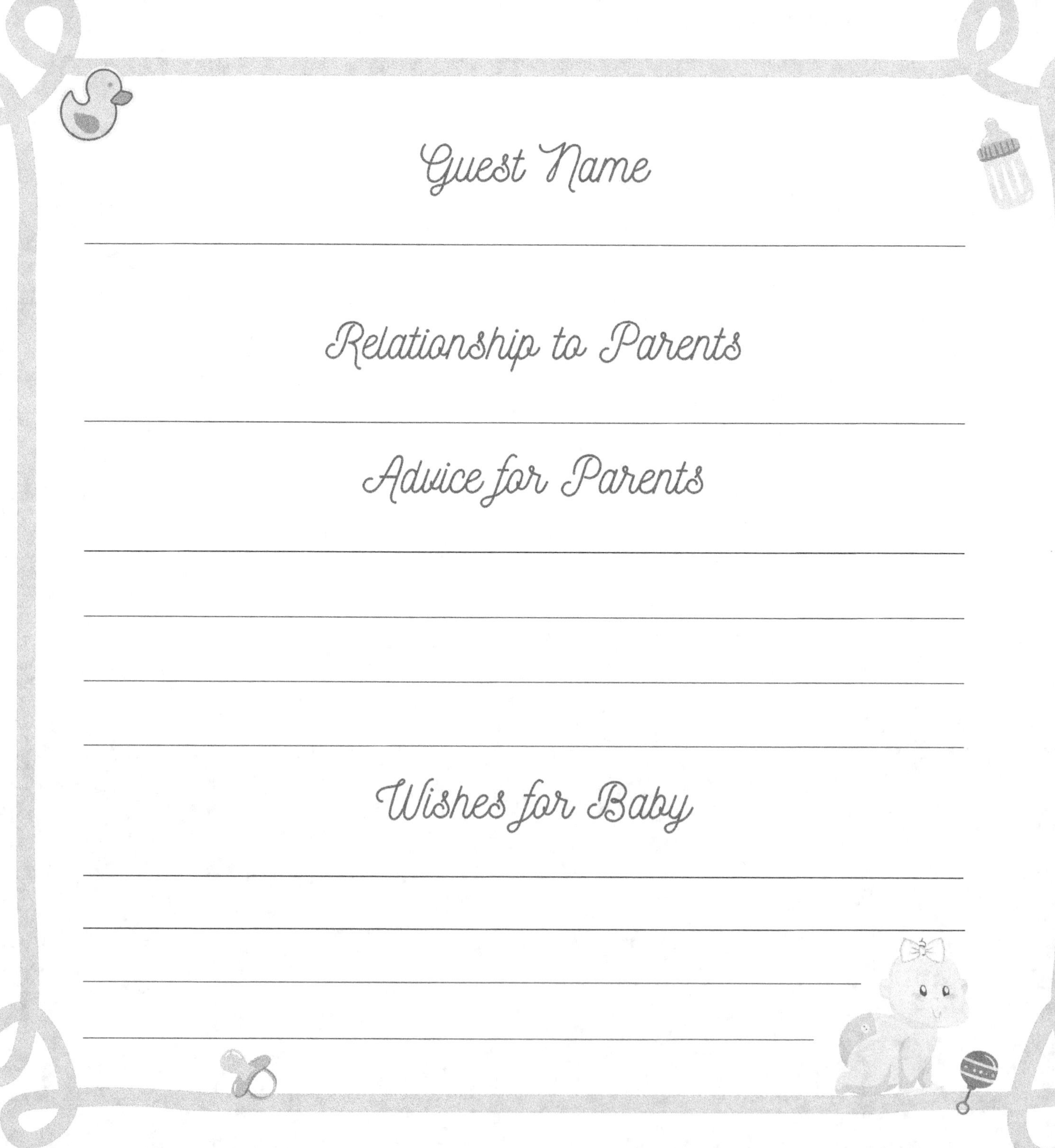
Guest Name

Relationship to Parents

Advice for Parents

Wishes for Baby

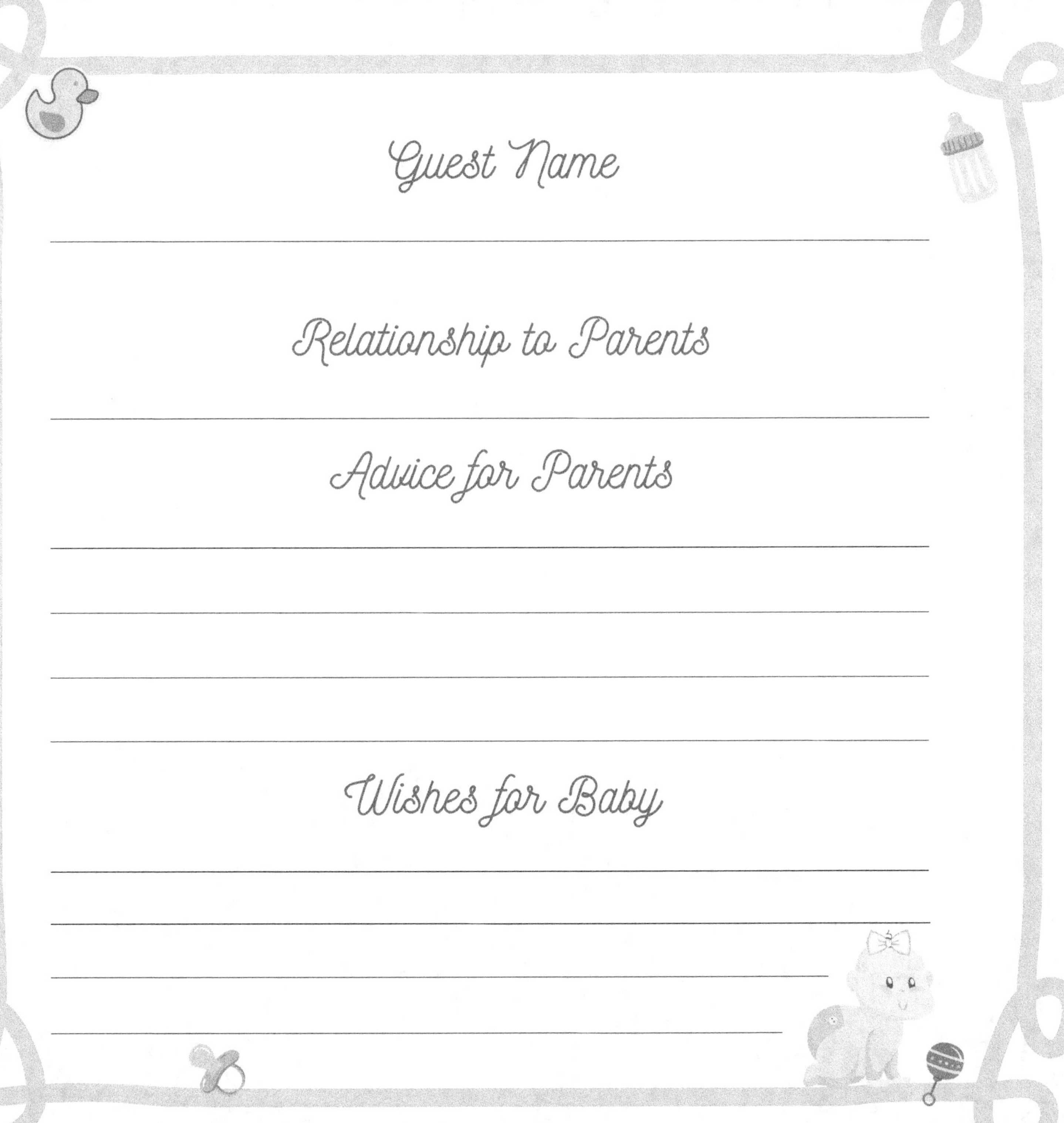

Guest Name

Relationship to Parents

Advice for Parents

Wishes for Baby

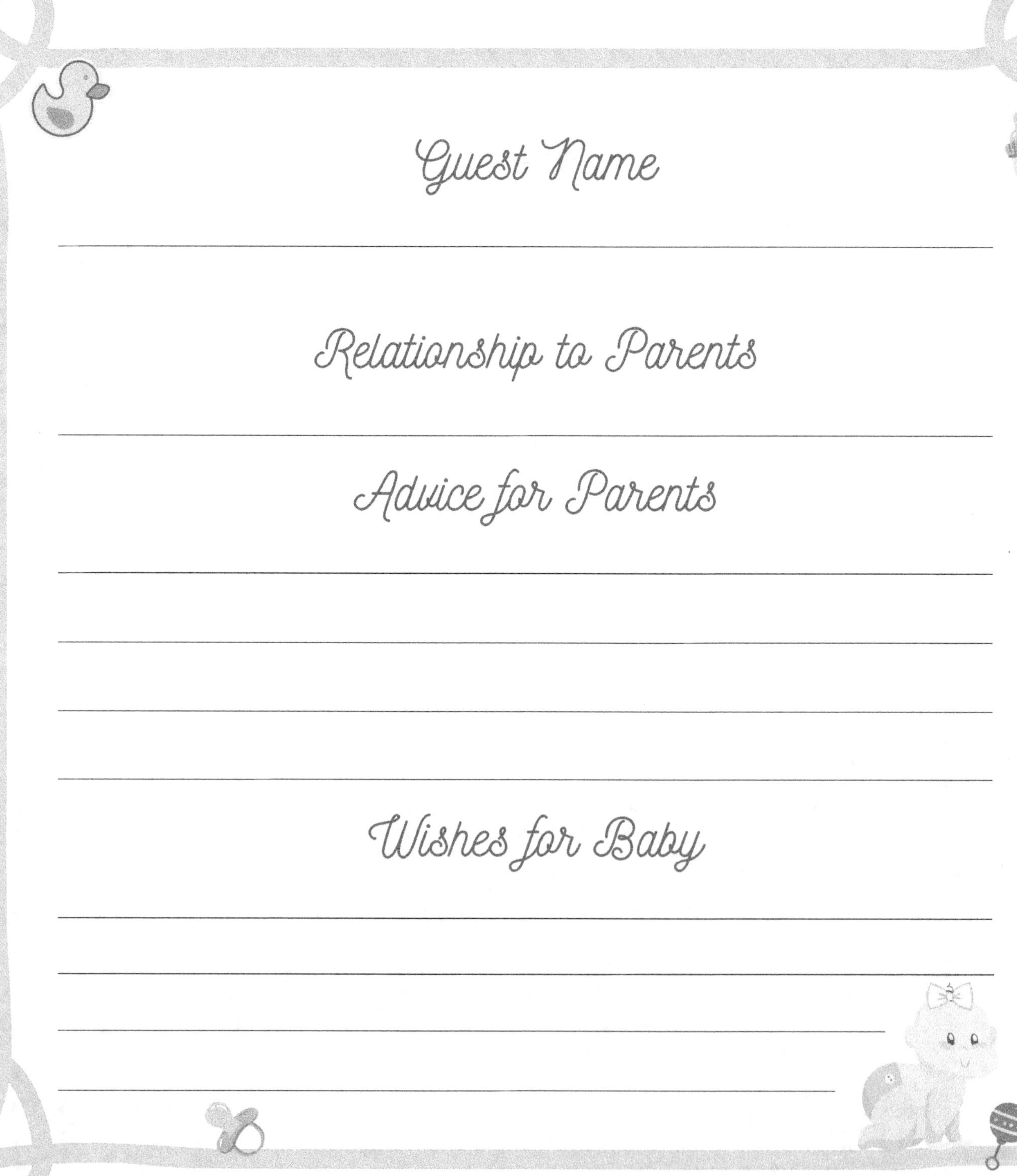

Guest Name

Relationship to Parents

Advice for Parents

Wishes for Baby

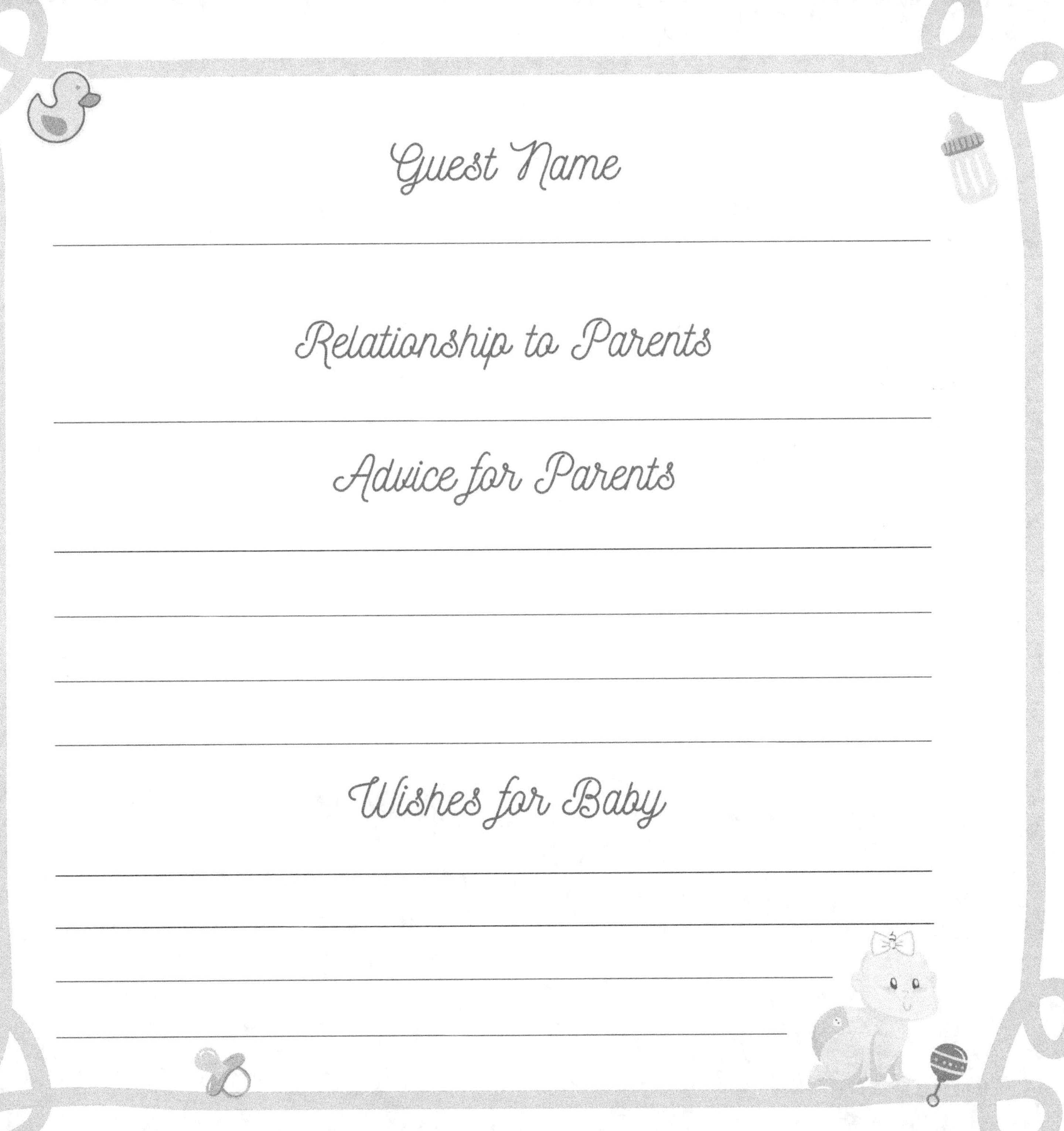

Guest Name

Relationship to Parents

Advice for Parents

Wishes for Baby

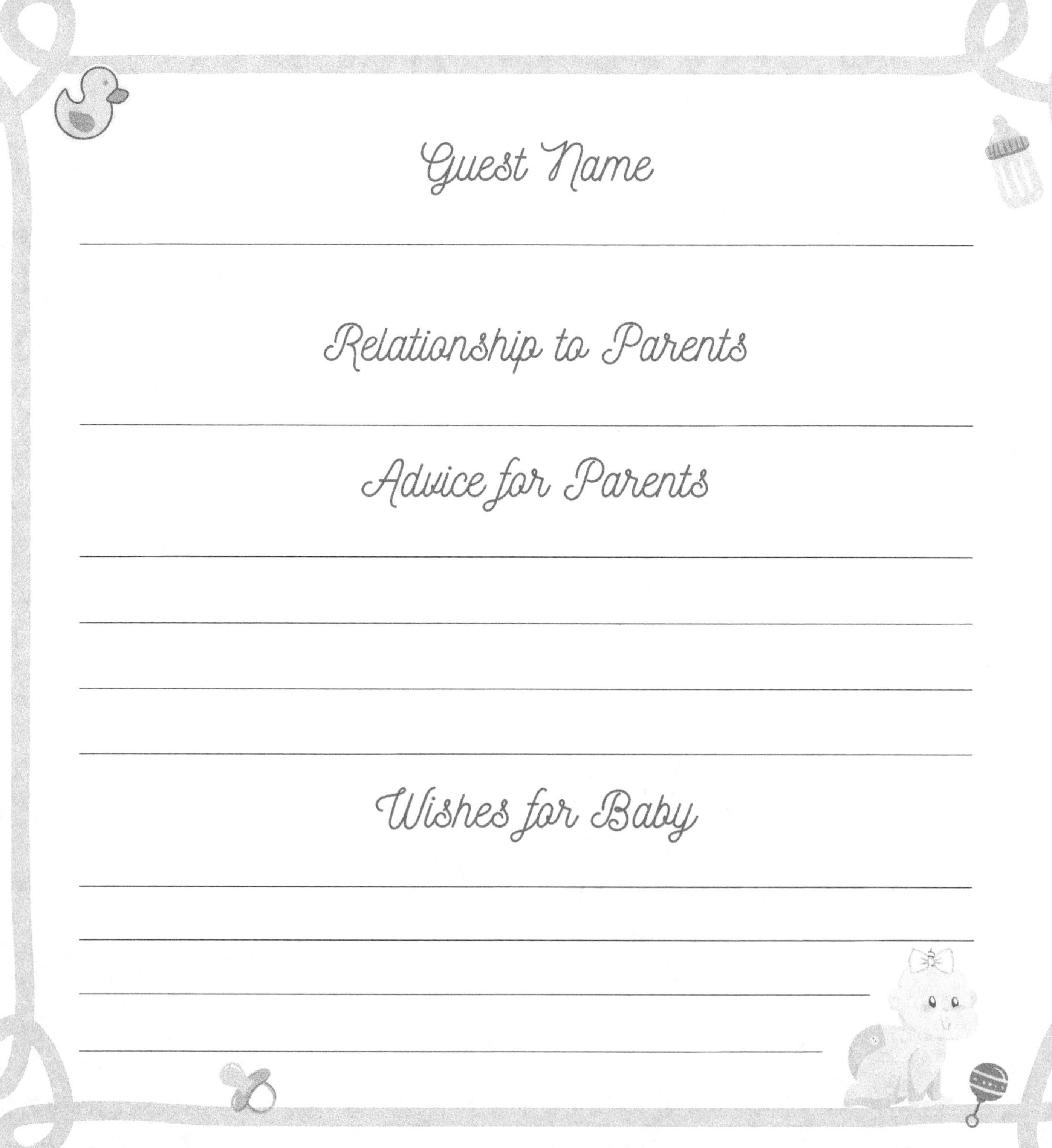

Guest Name

Relationship to Parents

Advice for Parents

Wishes for Baby

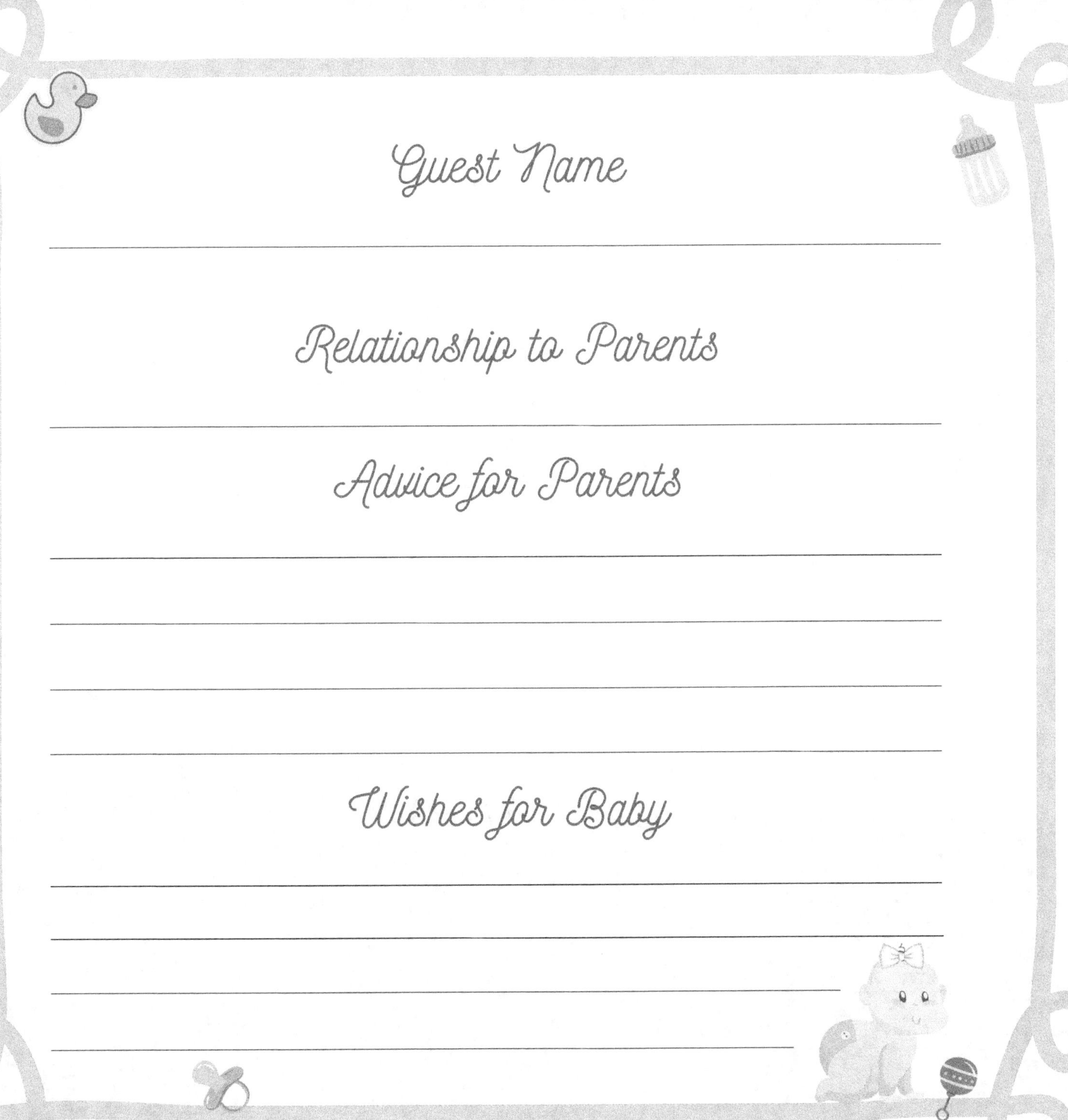

Guest Name

Relationship to Parents

Advice for Parents

Wishes for Baby

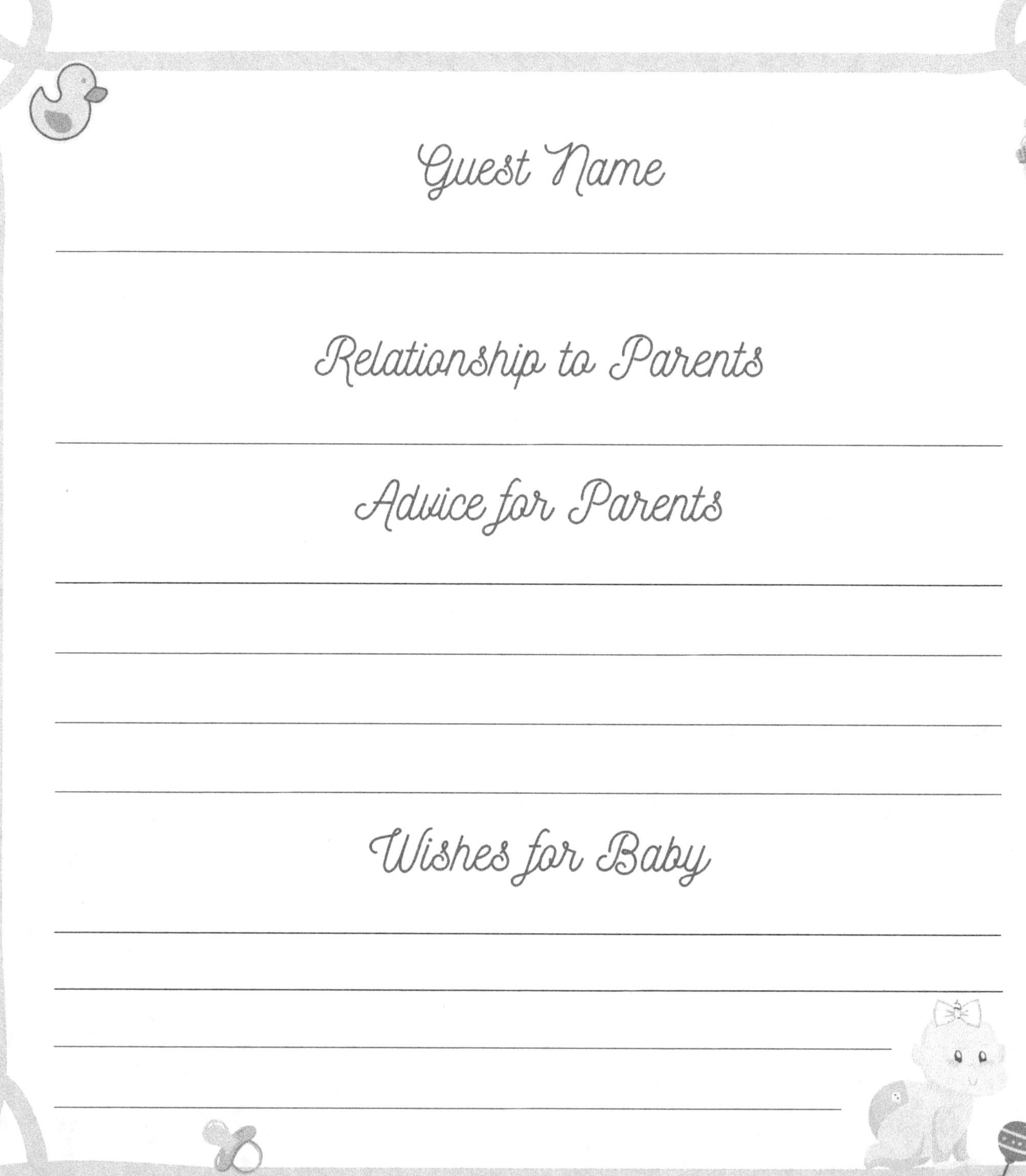

Guest Name

Relationship to Parents

Advice for Parents

Wishes for Baby

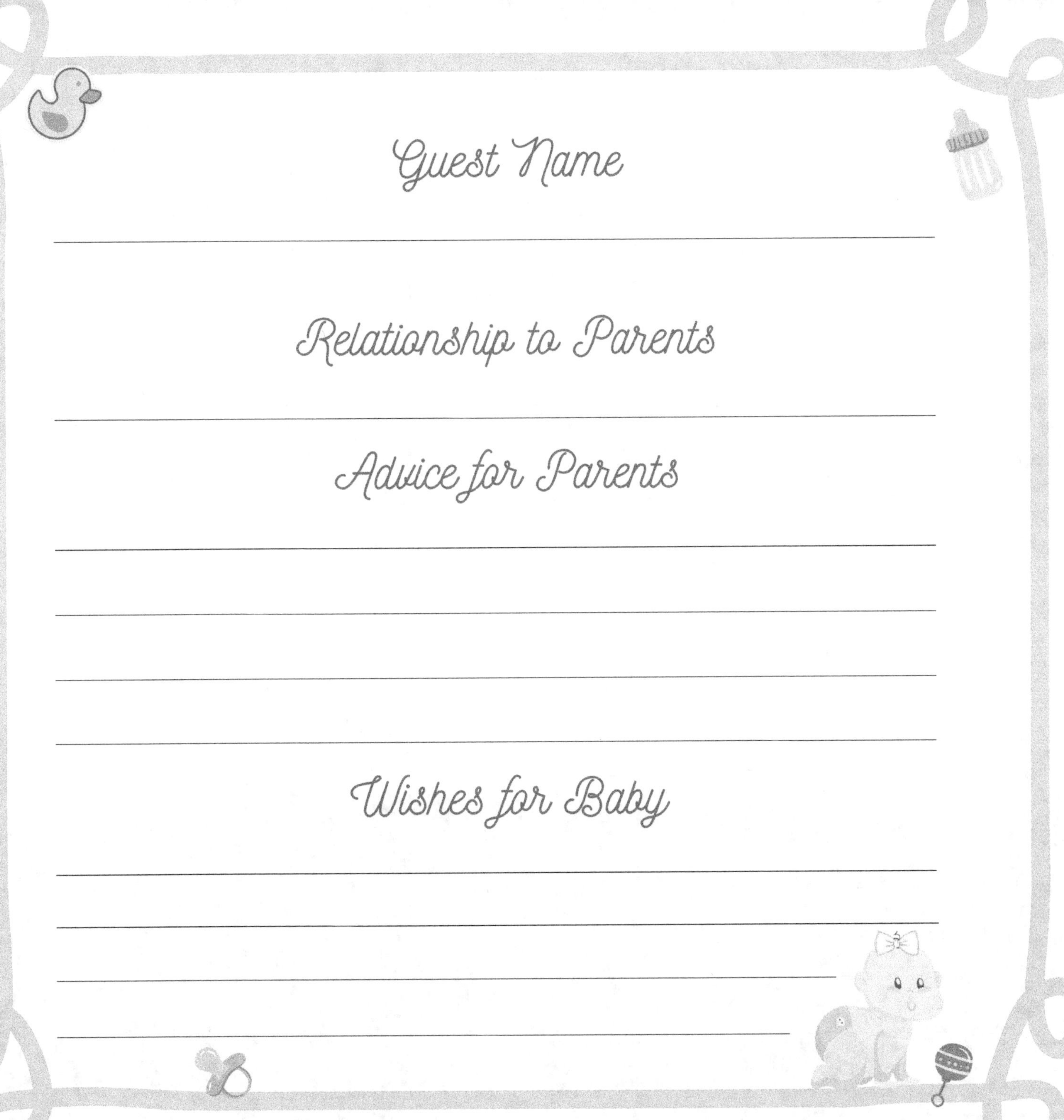Guest Name
Relationship to Parents
Advice for Parents
Wishes for Baby

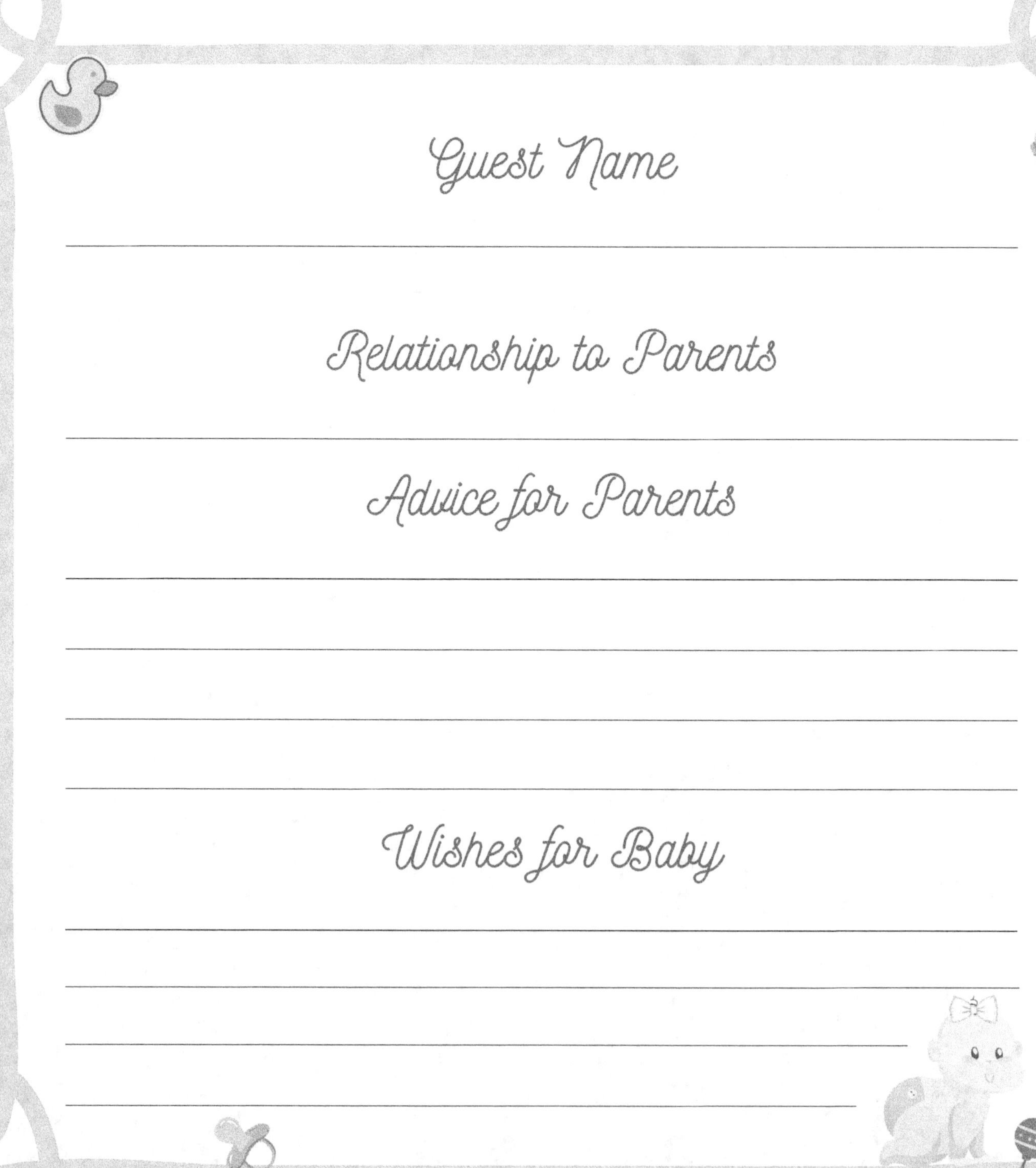

Guest Name

Relationship to Parents

Advice for Parents

Wishes for Baby

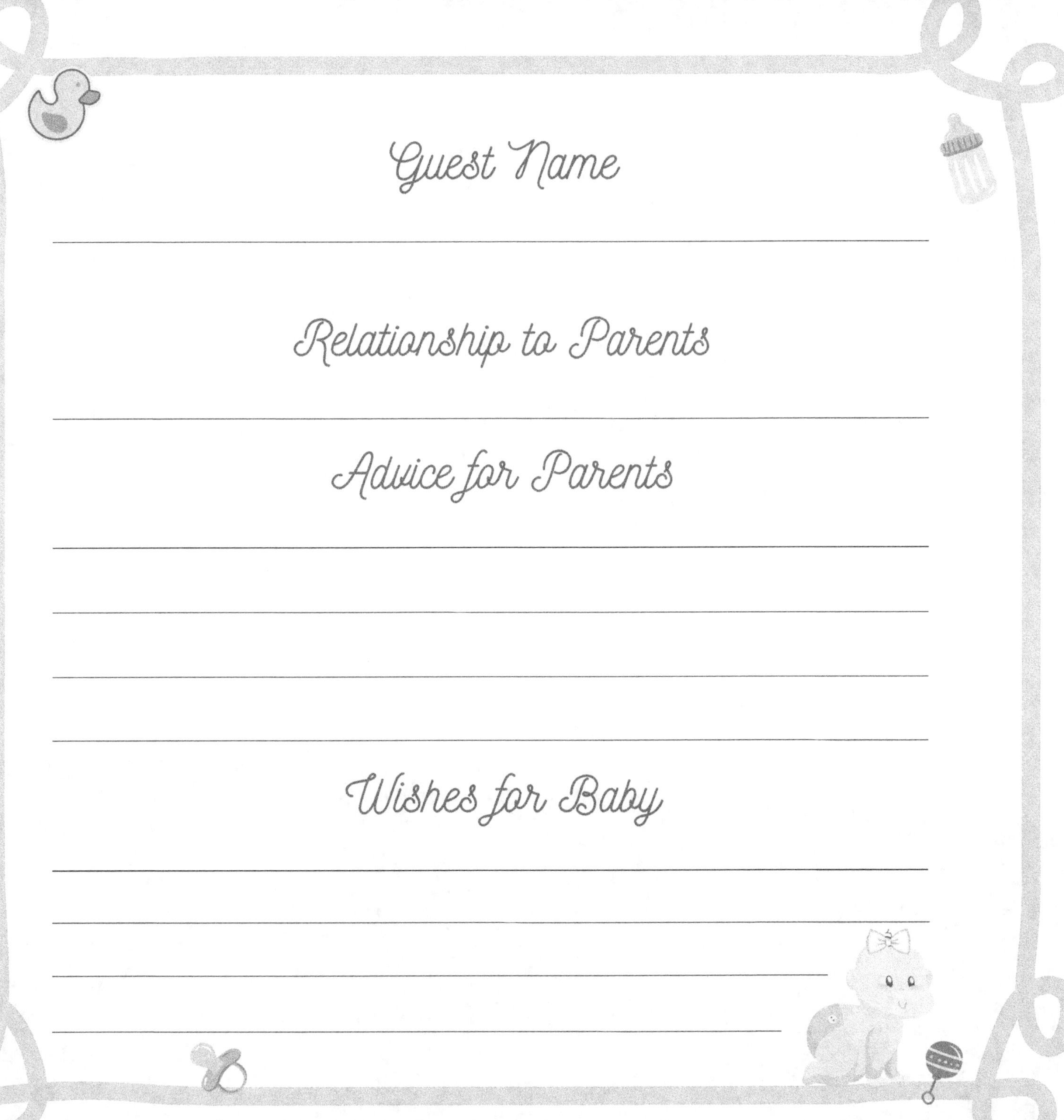
Guest Name

Relationship to Parents

Advice for Parents

Wishes for Baby

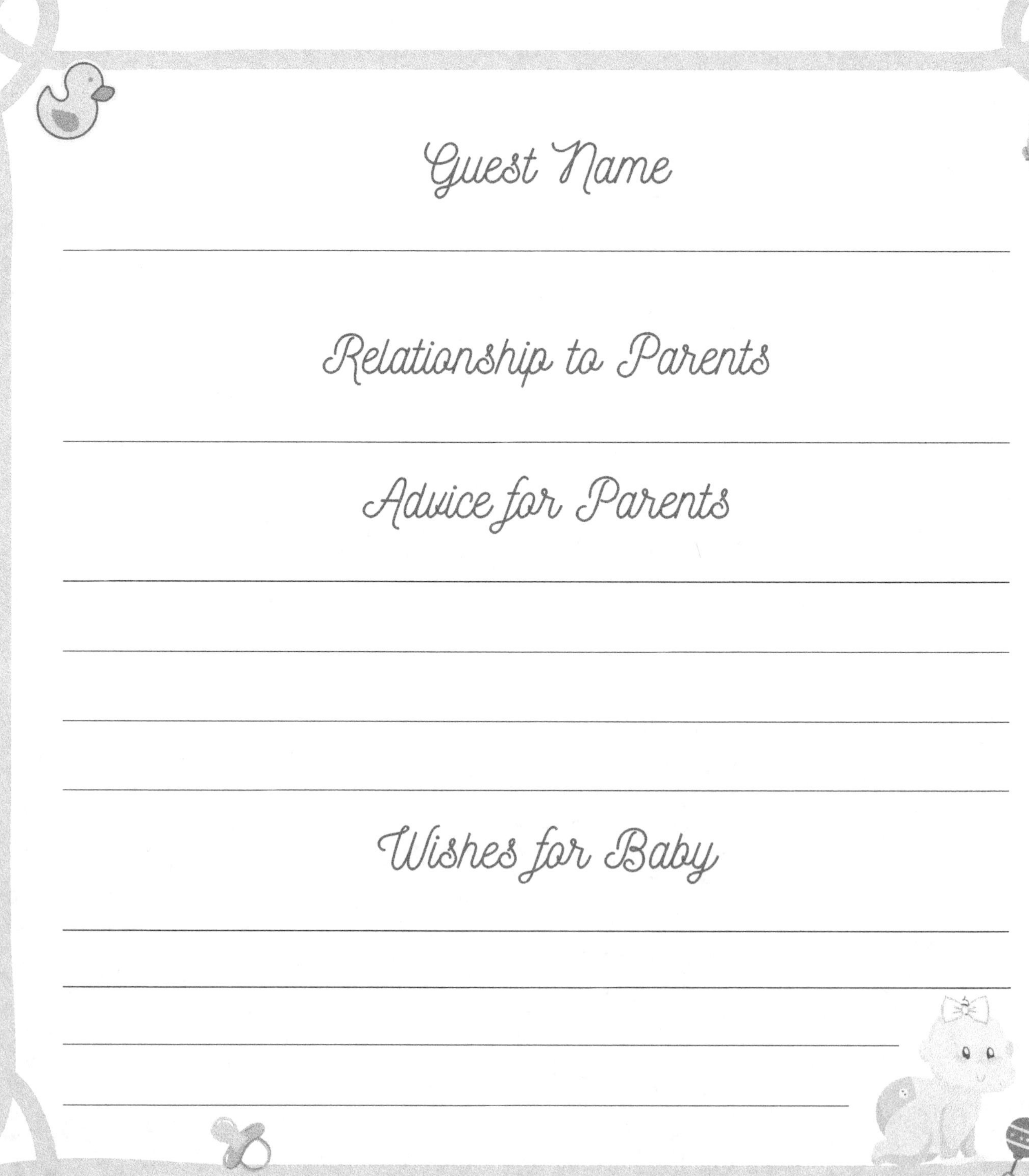

Guest Name

Relationship to Parents

Advice for Parents

Wishes for Baby

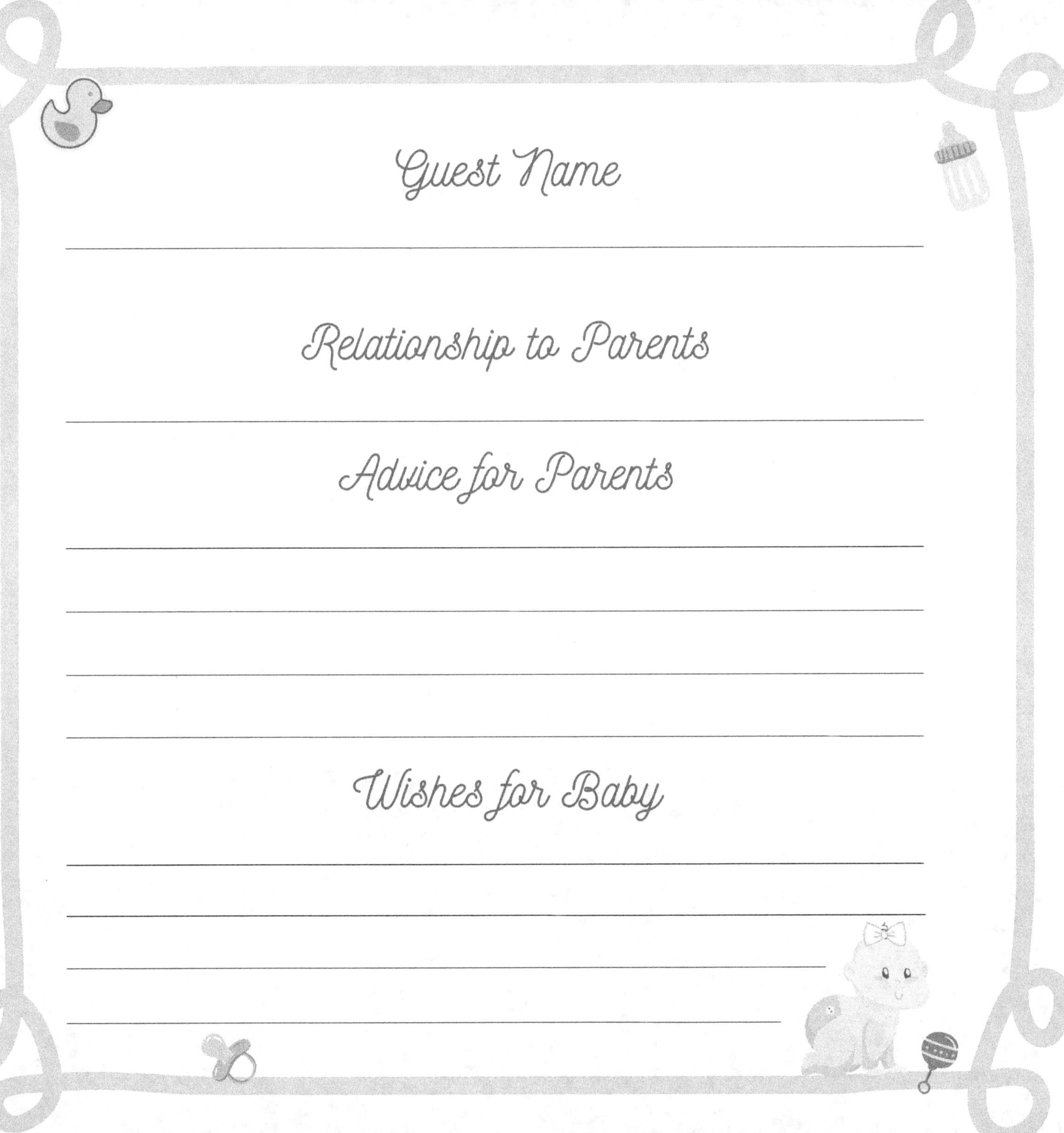

Guest Name

Relationship to Parents

Advice for Parents

Wishes for Baby

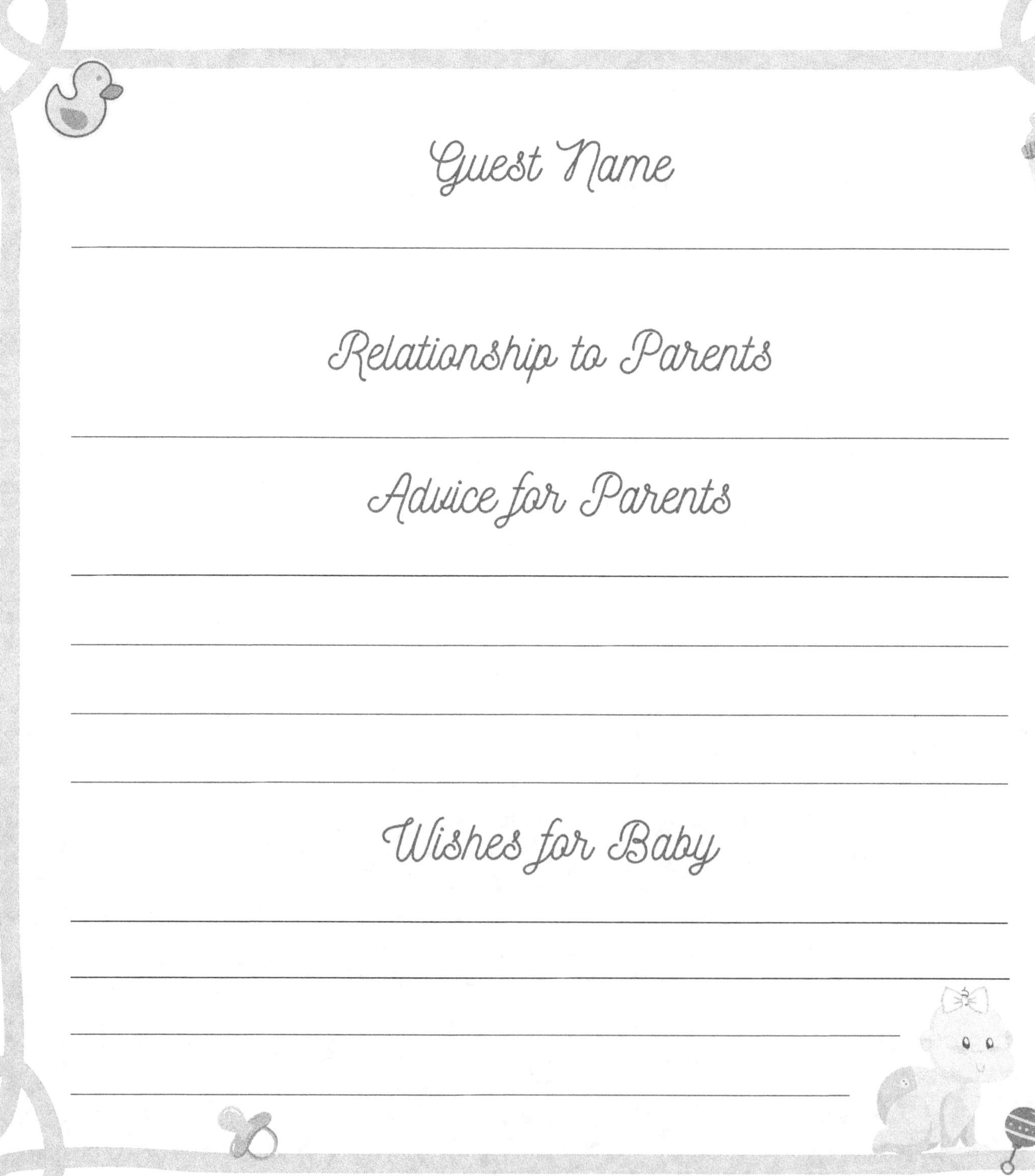

Guest Name
Relationship to Parents
Advice for Parents
Wishes for Baby

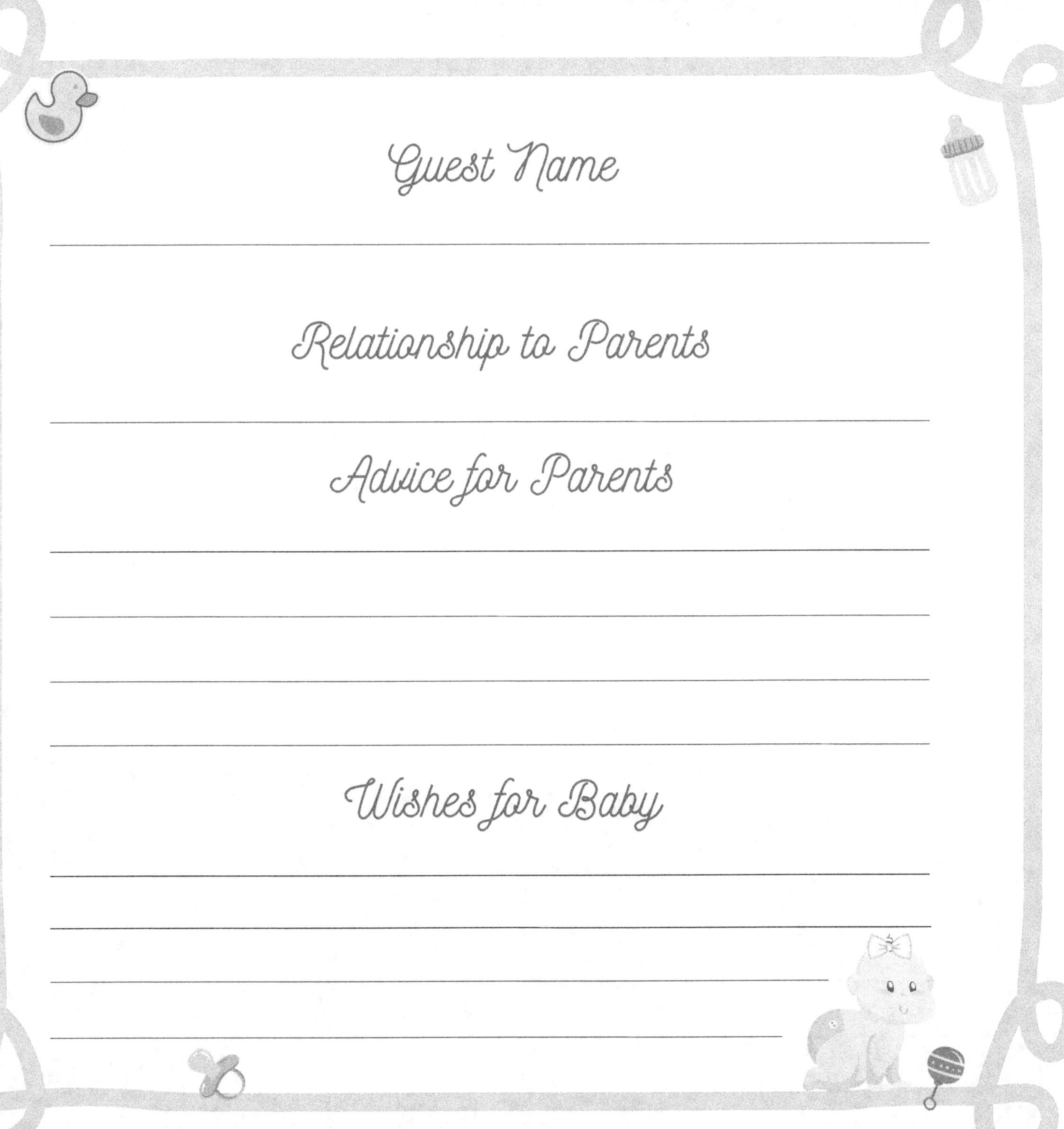

Guest Name
Relationship to Parents
Advice for Parents
Wishes for Baby

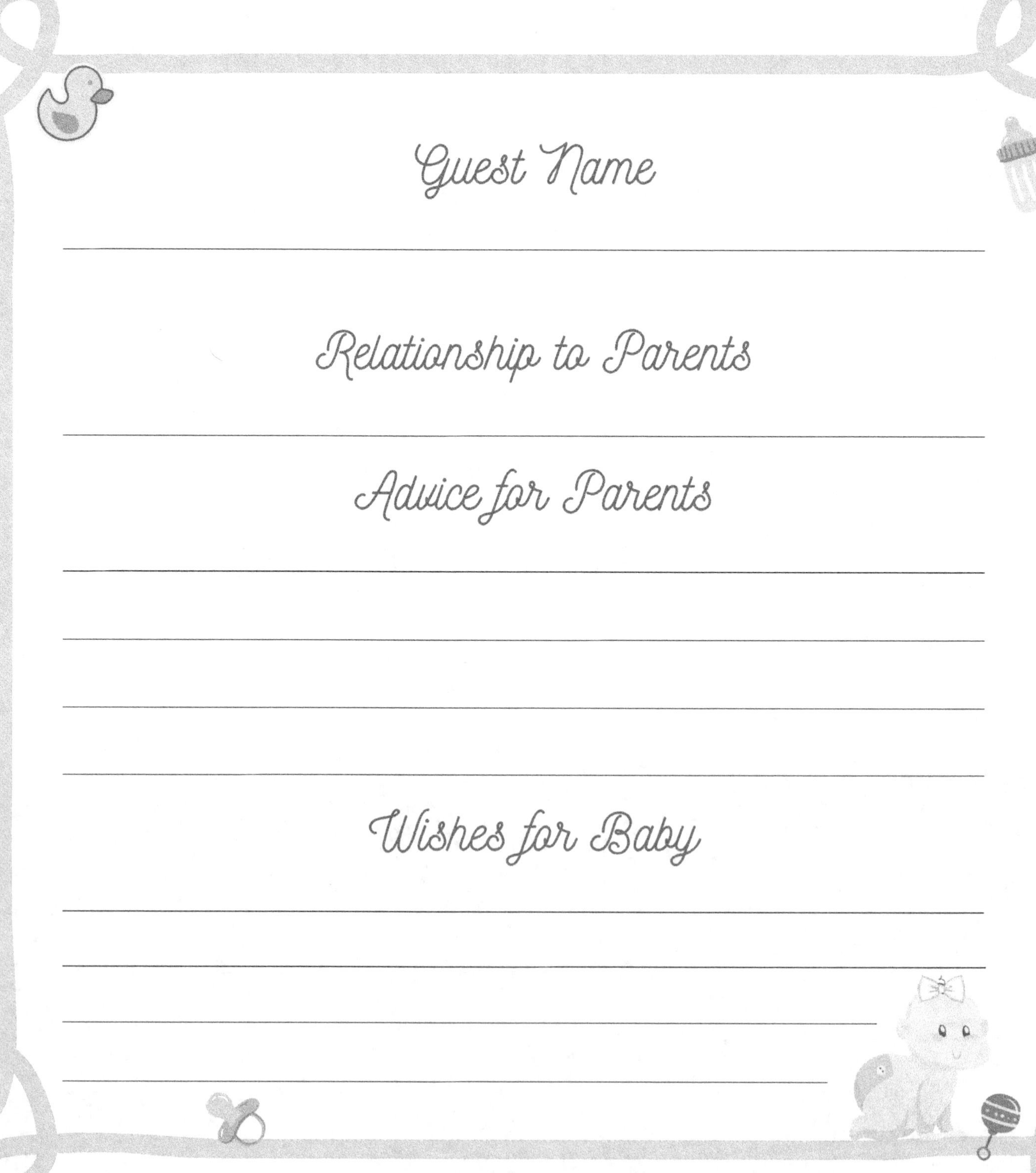Guest Name
Relationship to Parents
Advice for Parents
Wishes for Baby

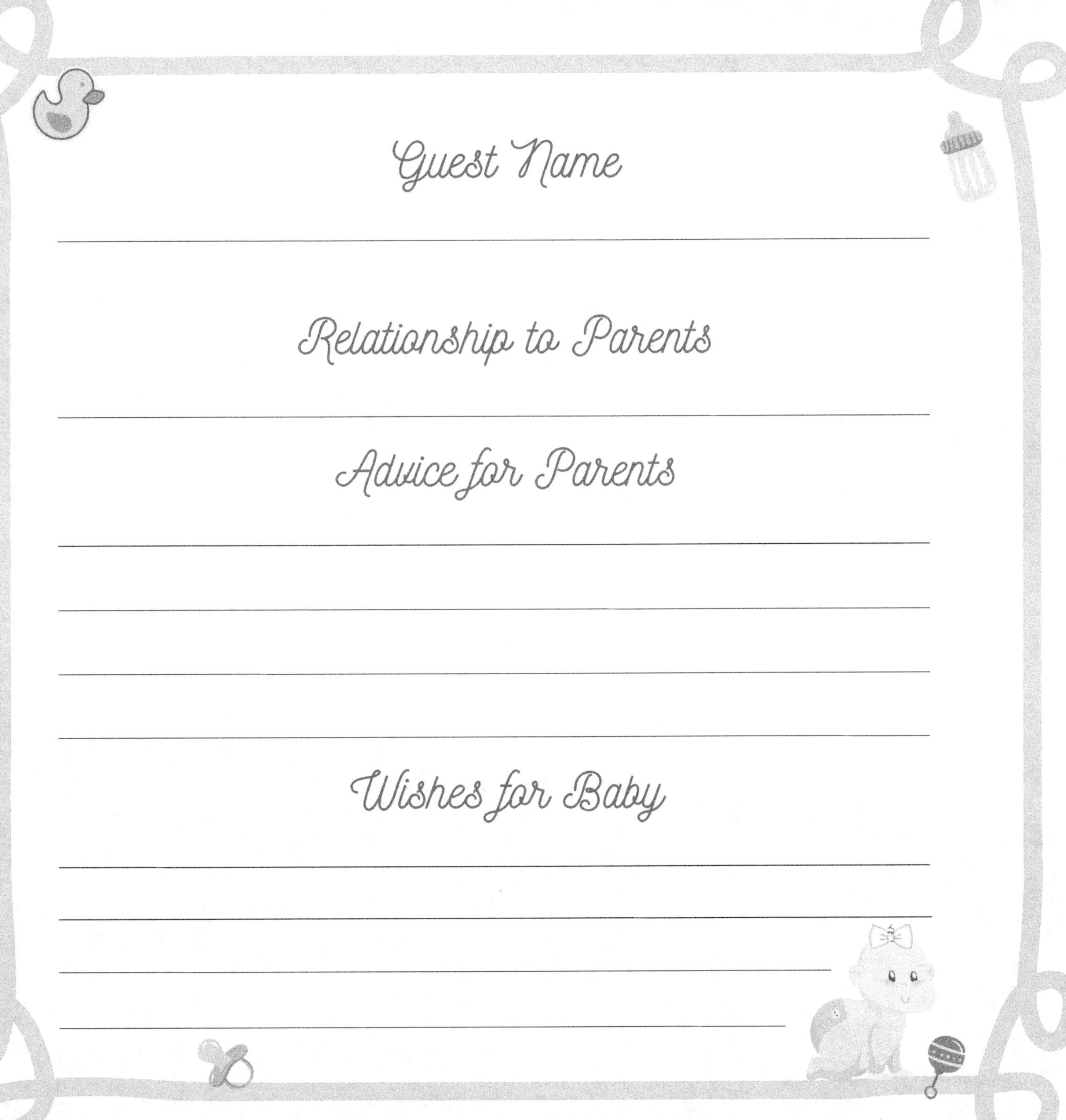

Guest Name

Relationship to Parents

Advice for Parents

Wishes for Baby

Guest Name

Relationship to Parents

Advice for Parents

Wishes for Baby

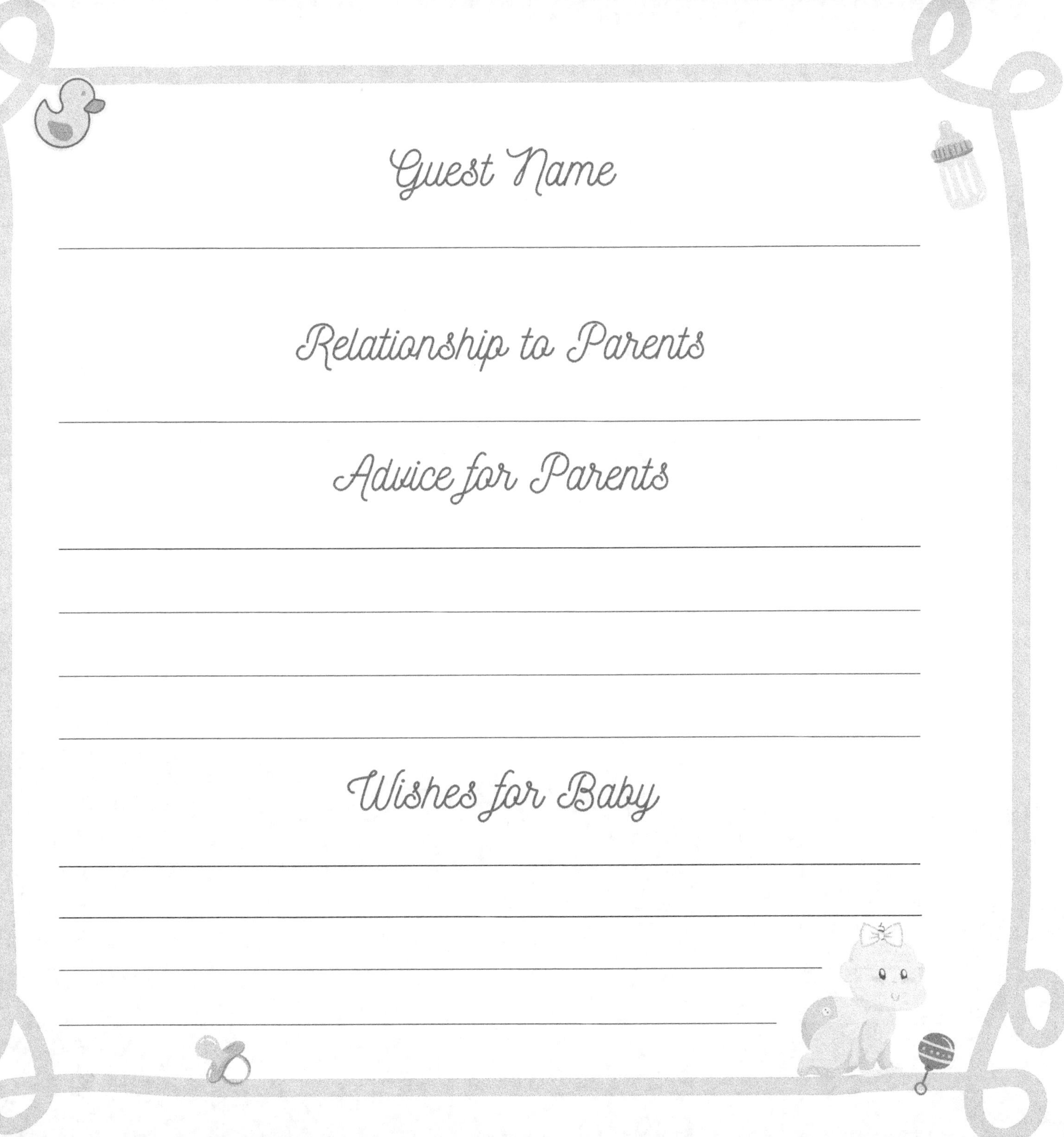

Guest Name

Relationship to Parents

Advice for Parents

Wishes for Baby

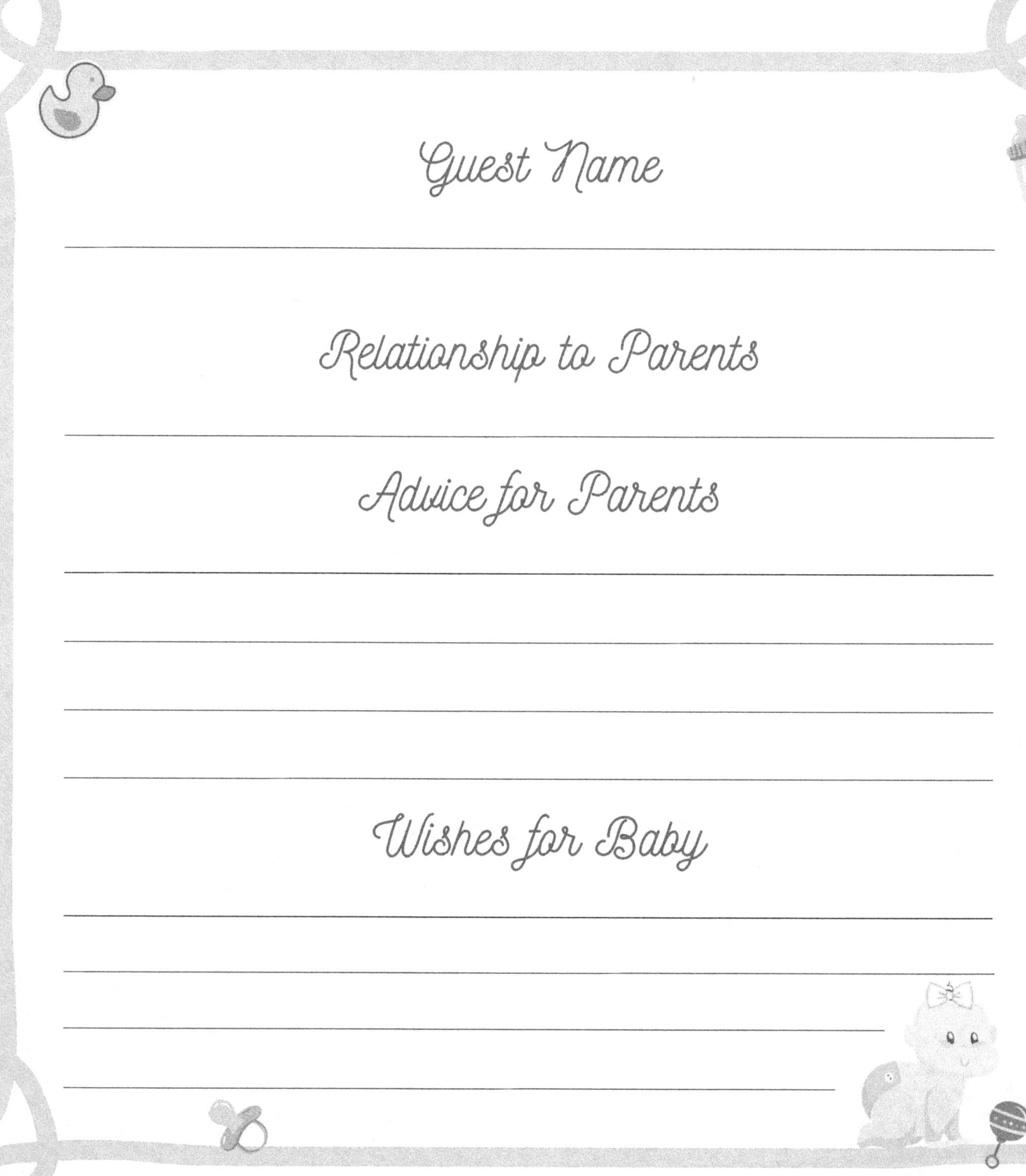

Guest Name

Relationship to Parents

Advice for Parents

Wishes for Baby

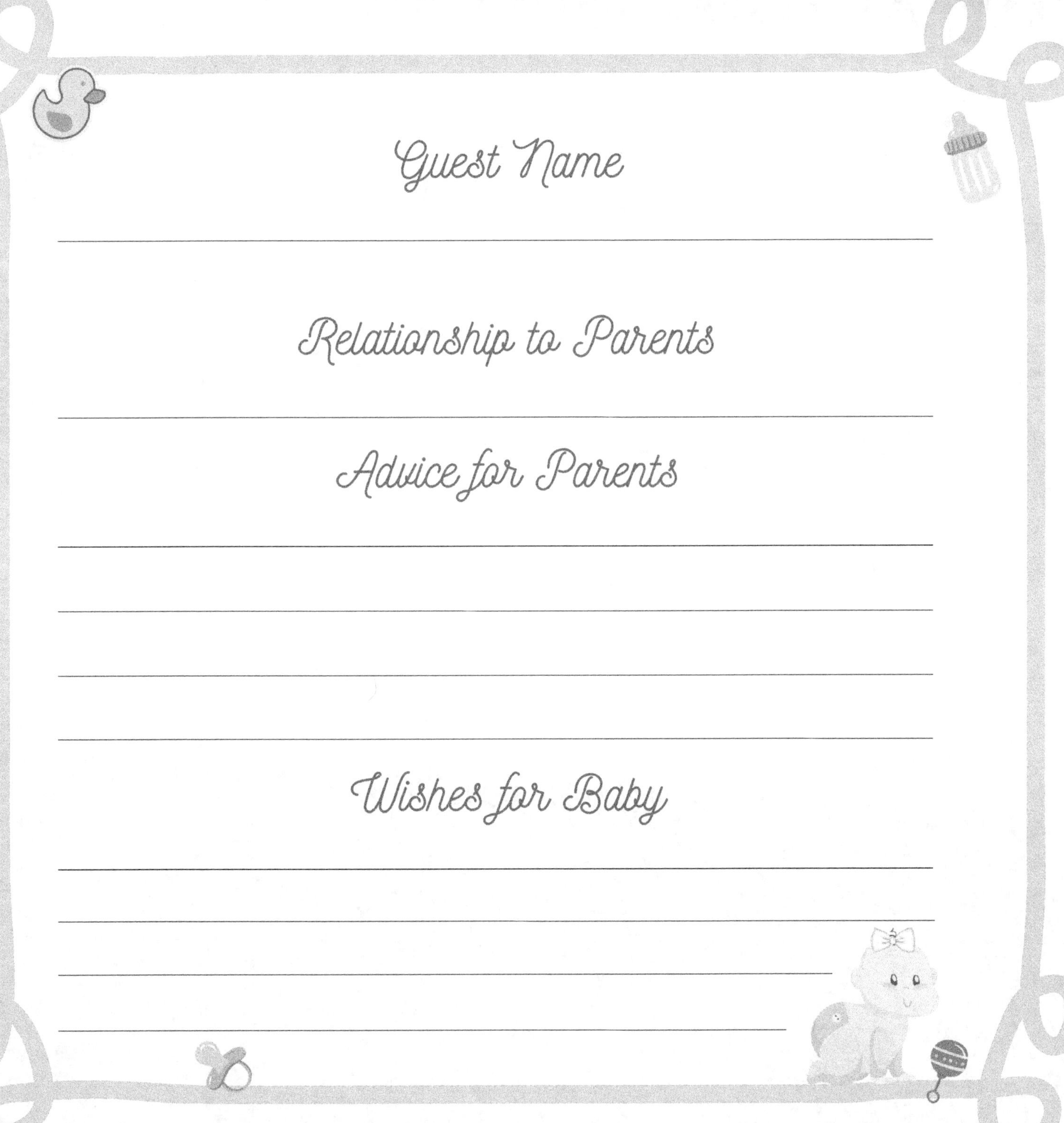

Guest Name

Relationship to Parents

Advice for Parents

Wishes for Baby

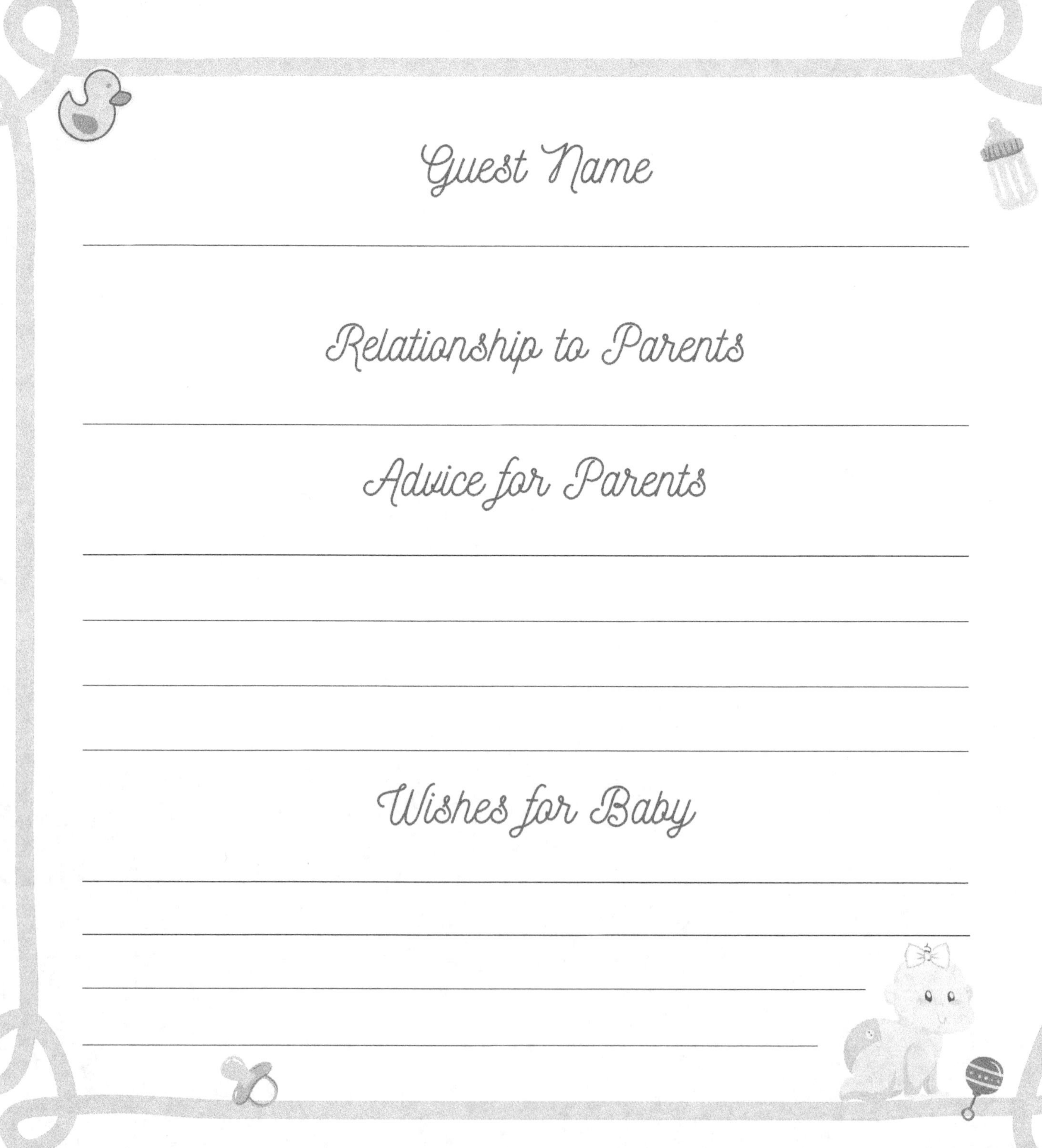

Guest Name
Relationship to Parents
Advice for Parents
Wishes for Baby

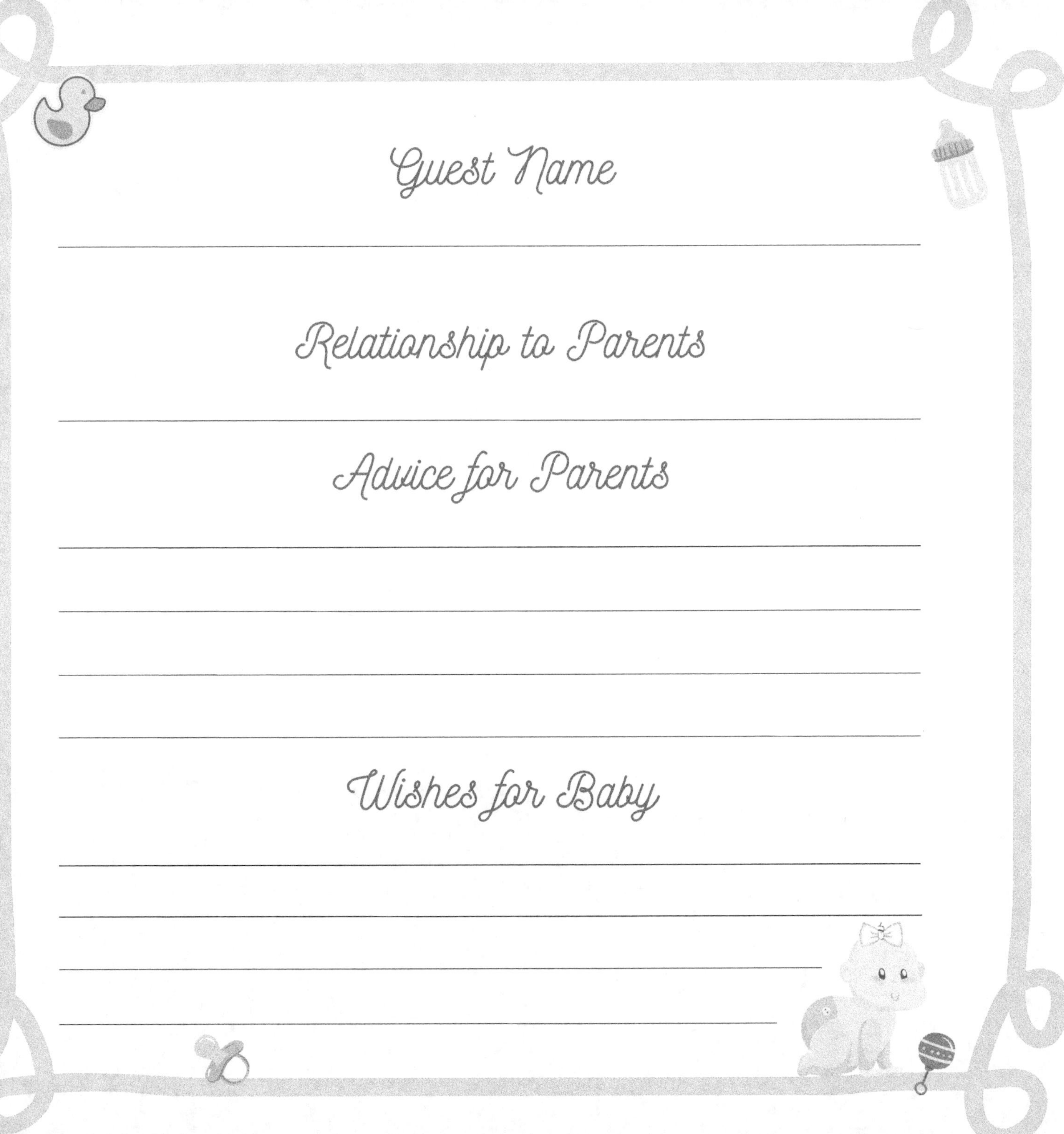

Guest Name

Relationship to Parents

Advice for Parents

Wishes for Baby

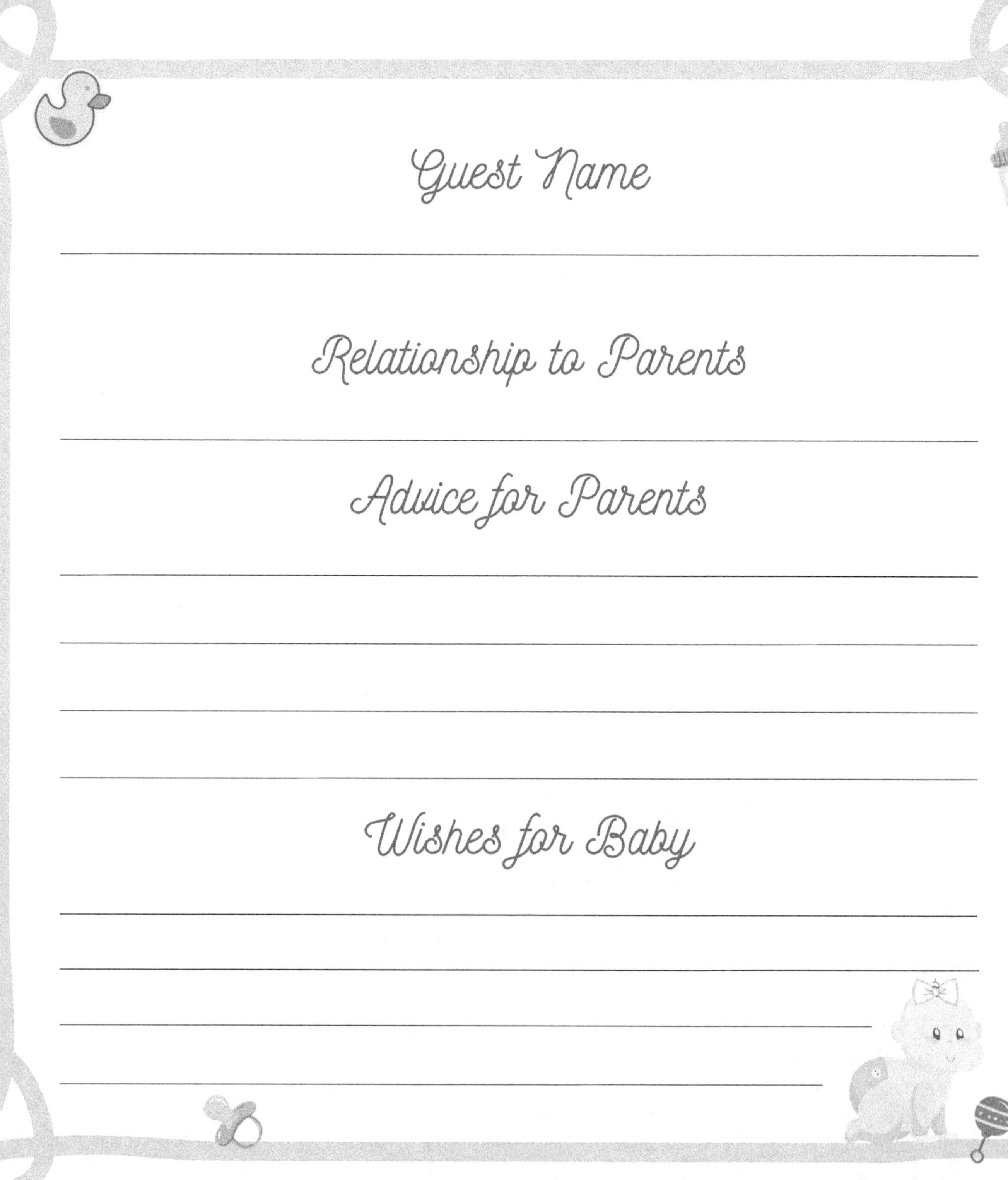
Guest Name

Relationship to Parents

Advice for Parents

Wishes for Baby

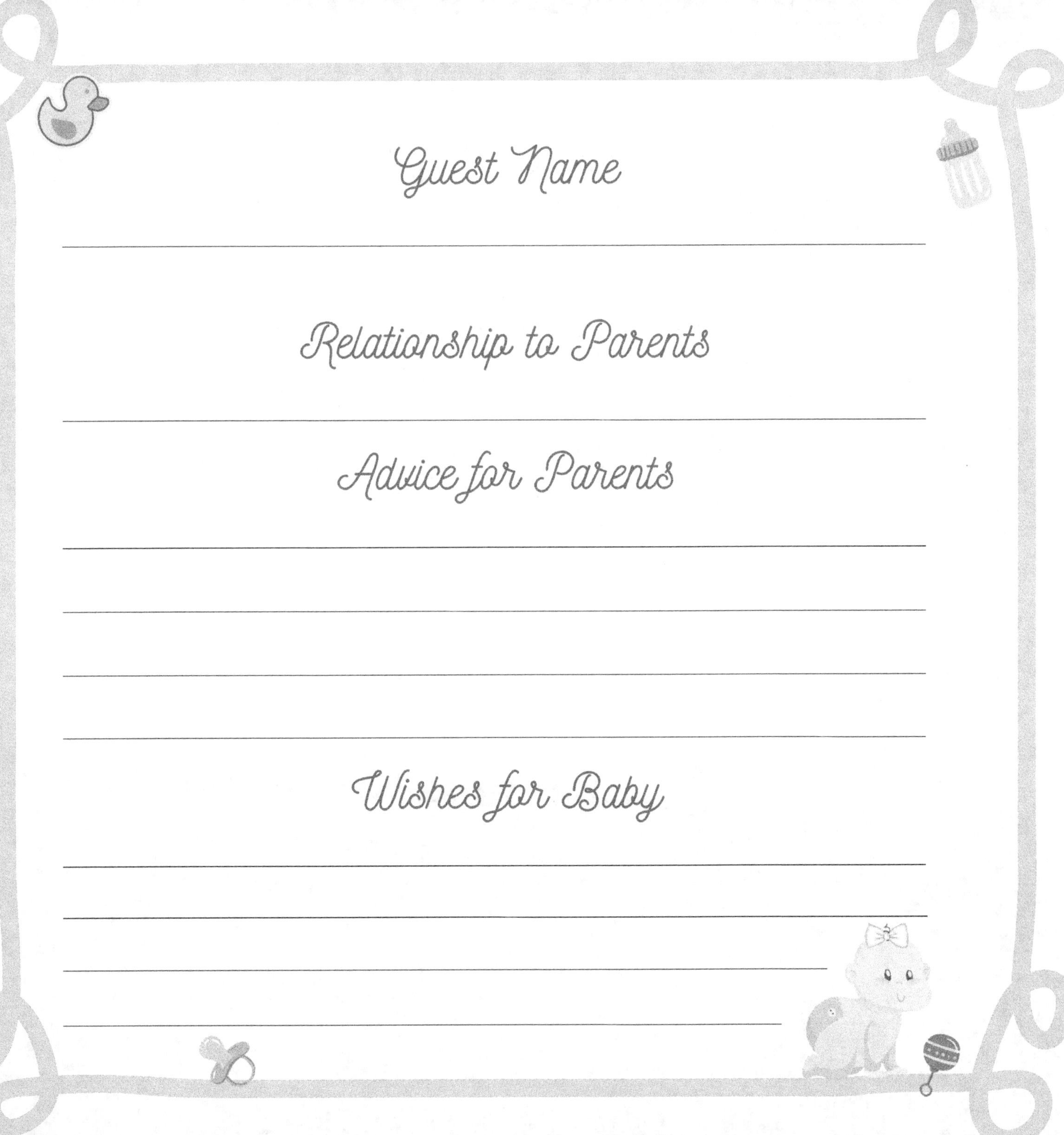

Guest Name

Relationship to Parents

Advice for Parents

Wishes for Baby

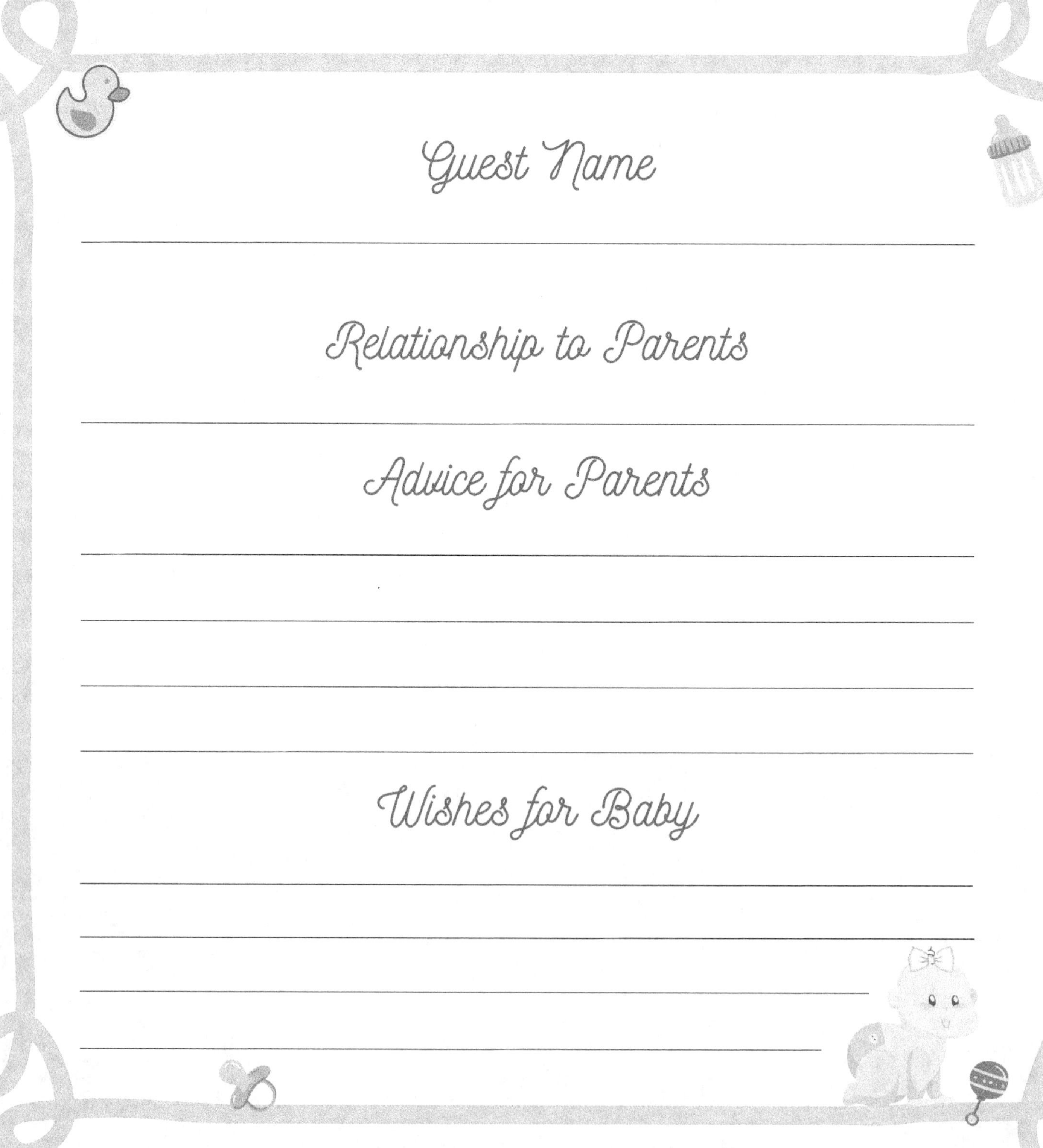
Guest Name
Relationship to Parents
Advice for Parents
Wishes for Baby

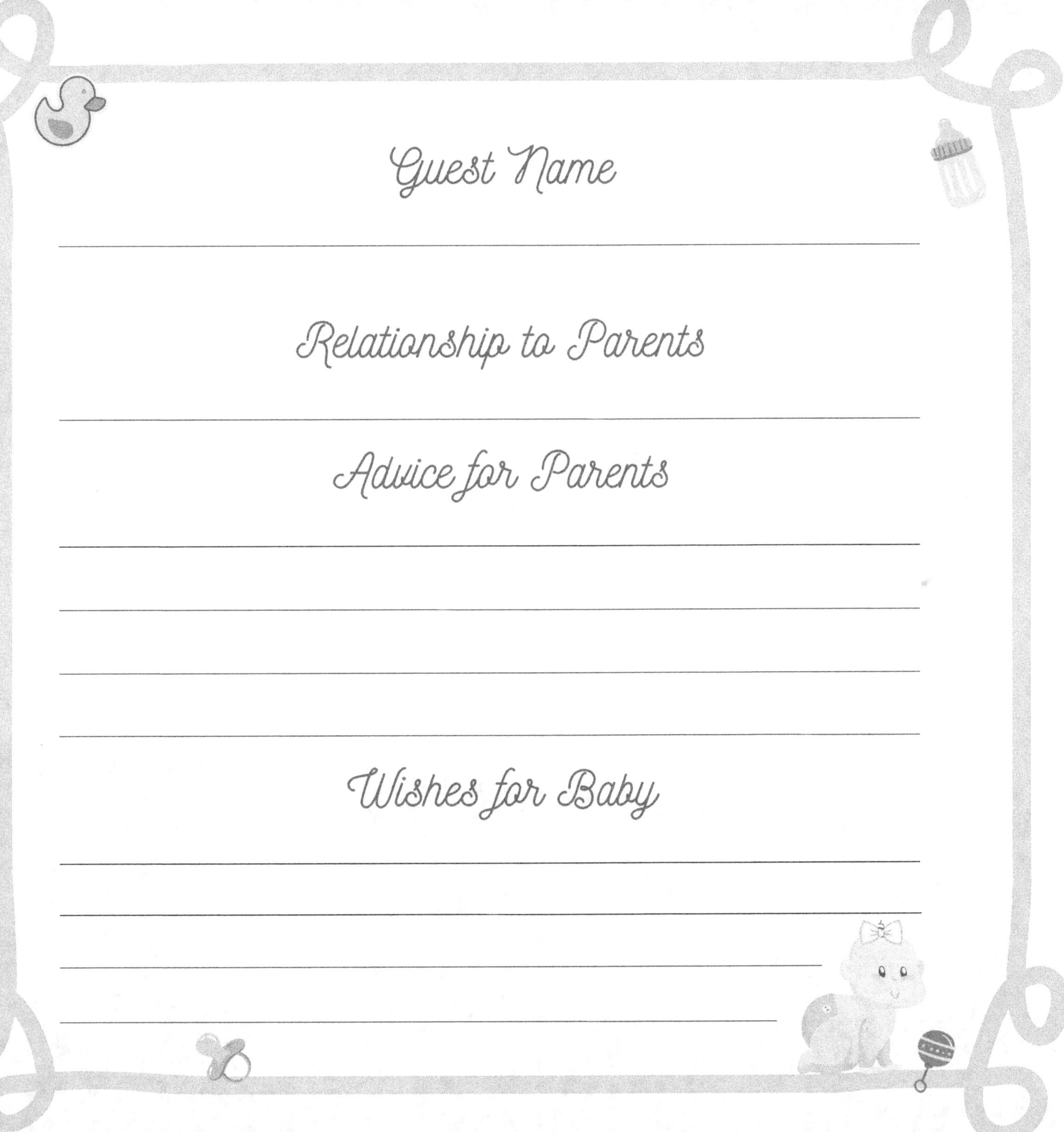

Guest Name

Relationship to Parents

Advice for Parents

Wishes for Baby

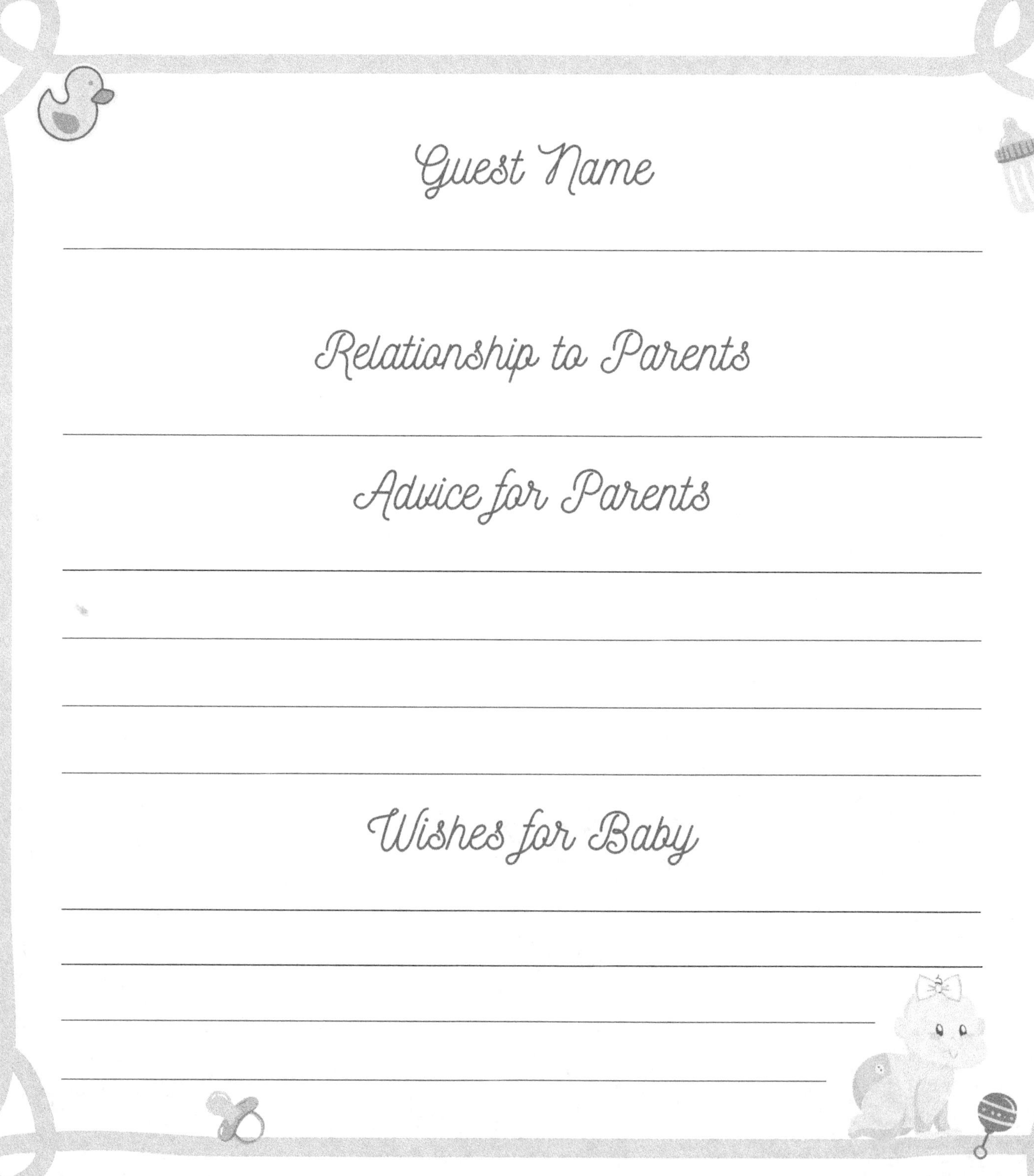

Guest Name

Relationship to Parents

Advice for Parents

Wishes for Baby

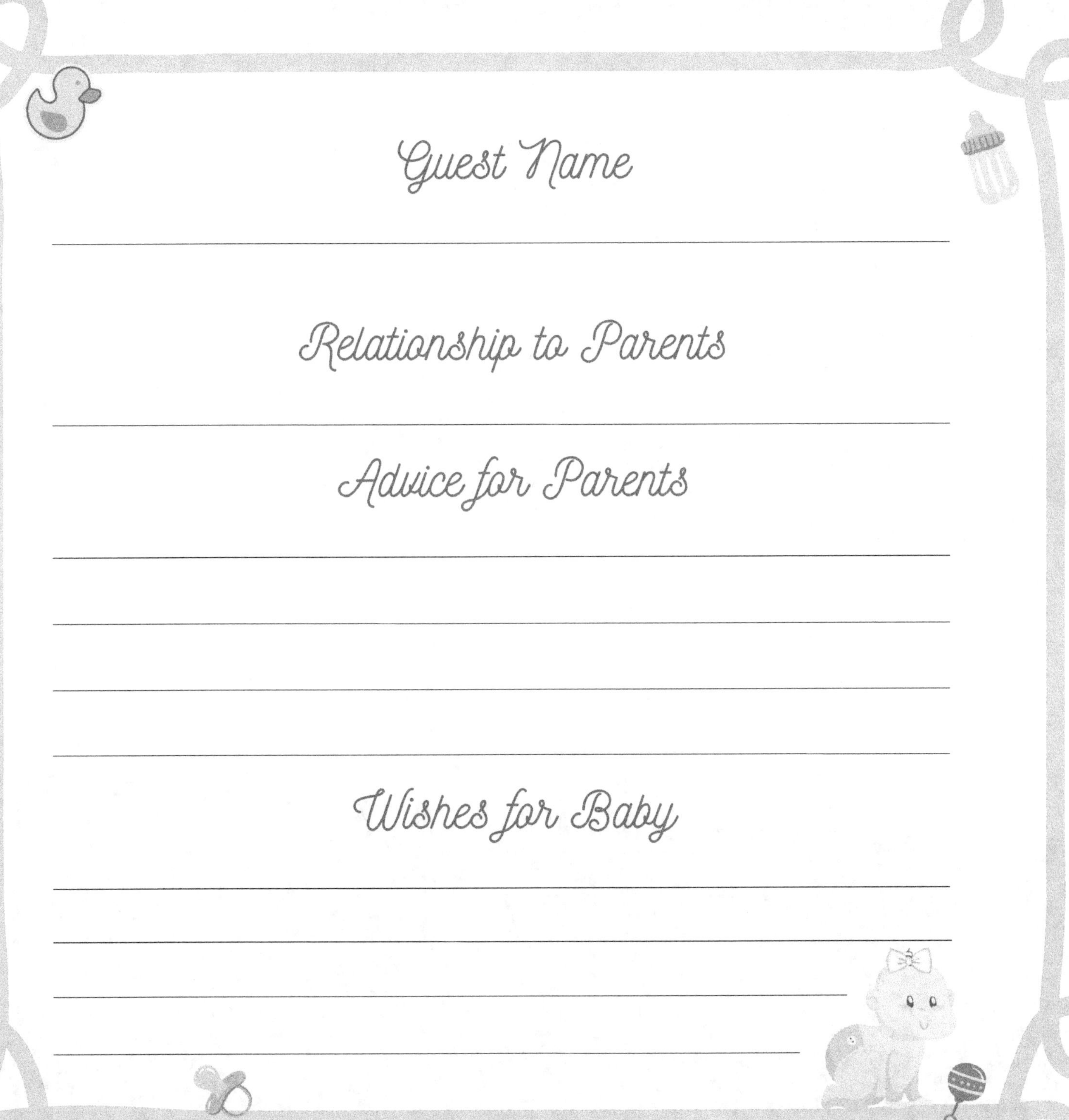

Guest Name

Relationship to Parents

Advice for Parents

Wishes for Baby

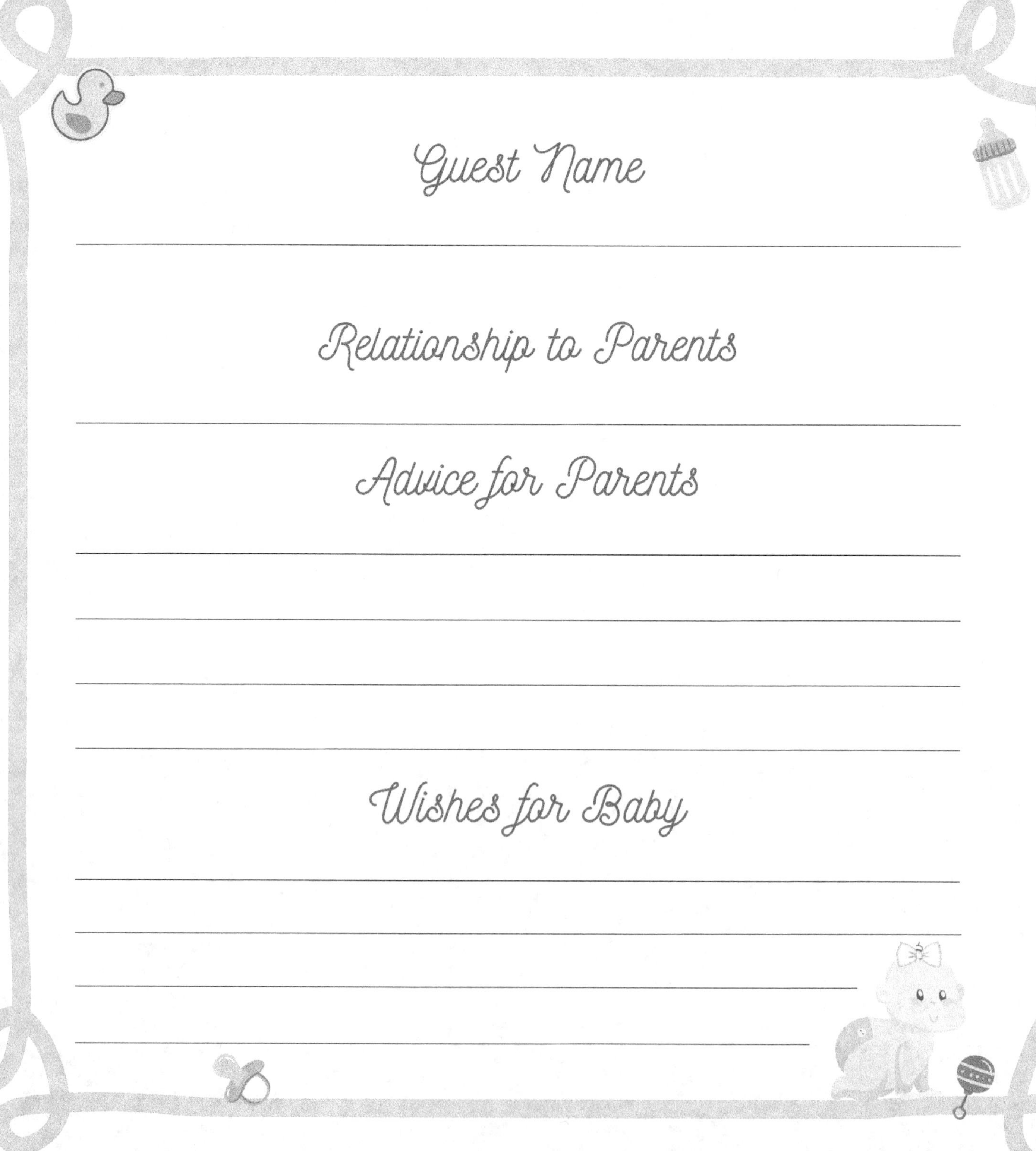
Guest Name

Relationship to Parents

Advice for Parents

Wishes for Baby

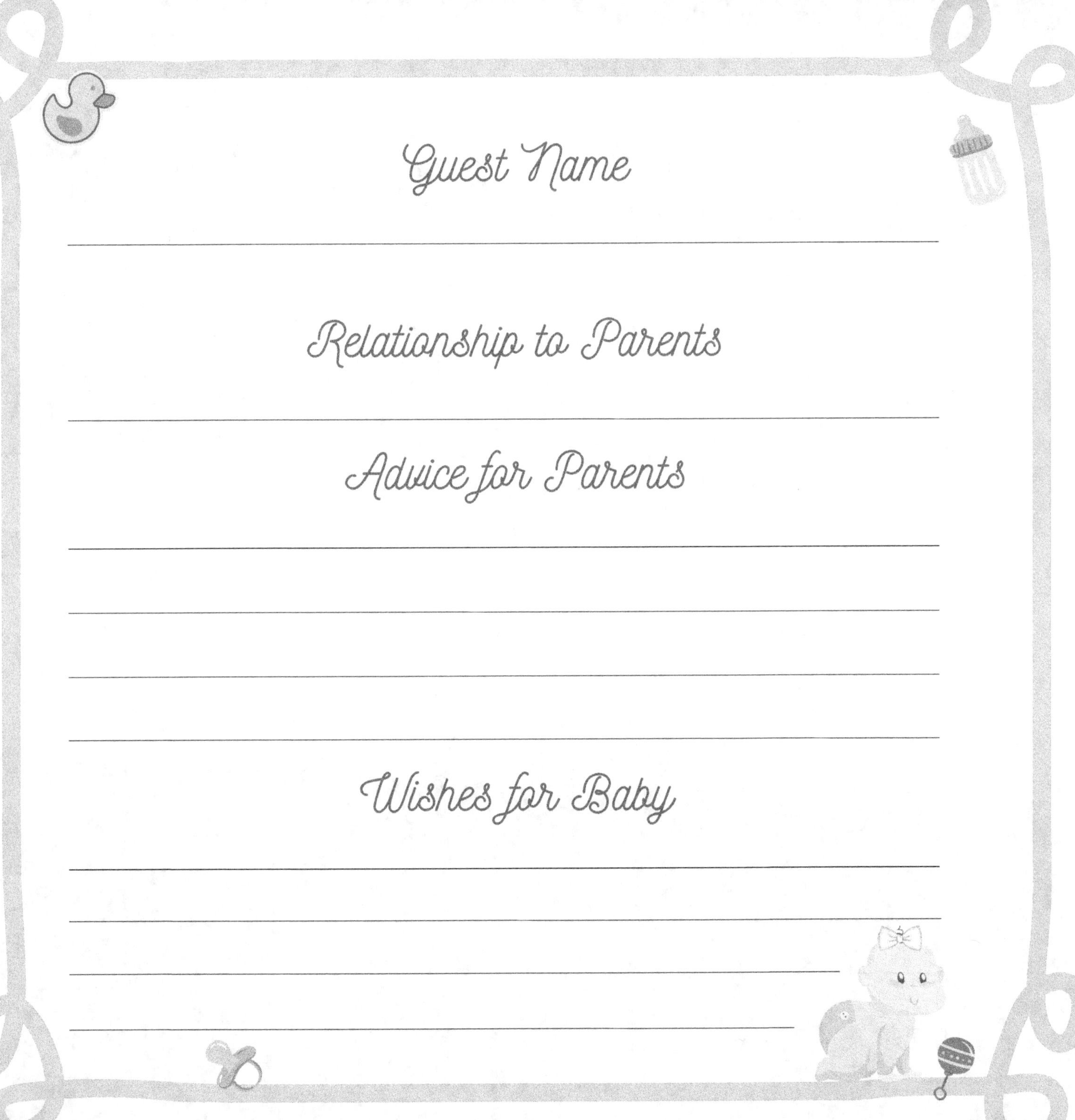

Guest Name

____

Relationship to Parents

____

Advice for Parents

____

____

____

____

Wishes for Baby

____

____

____

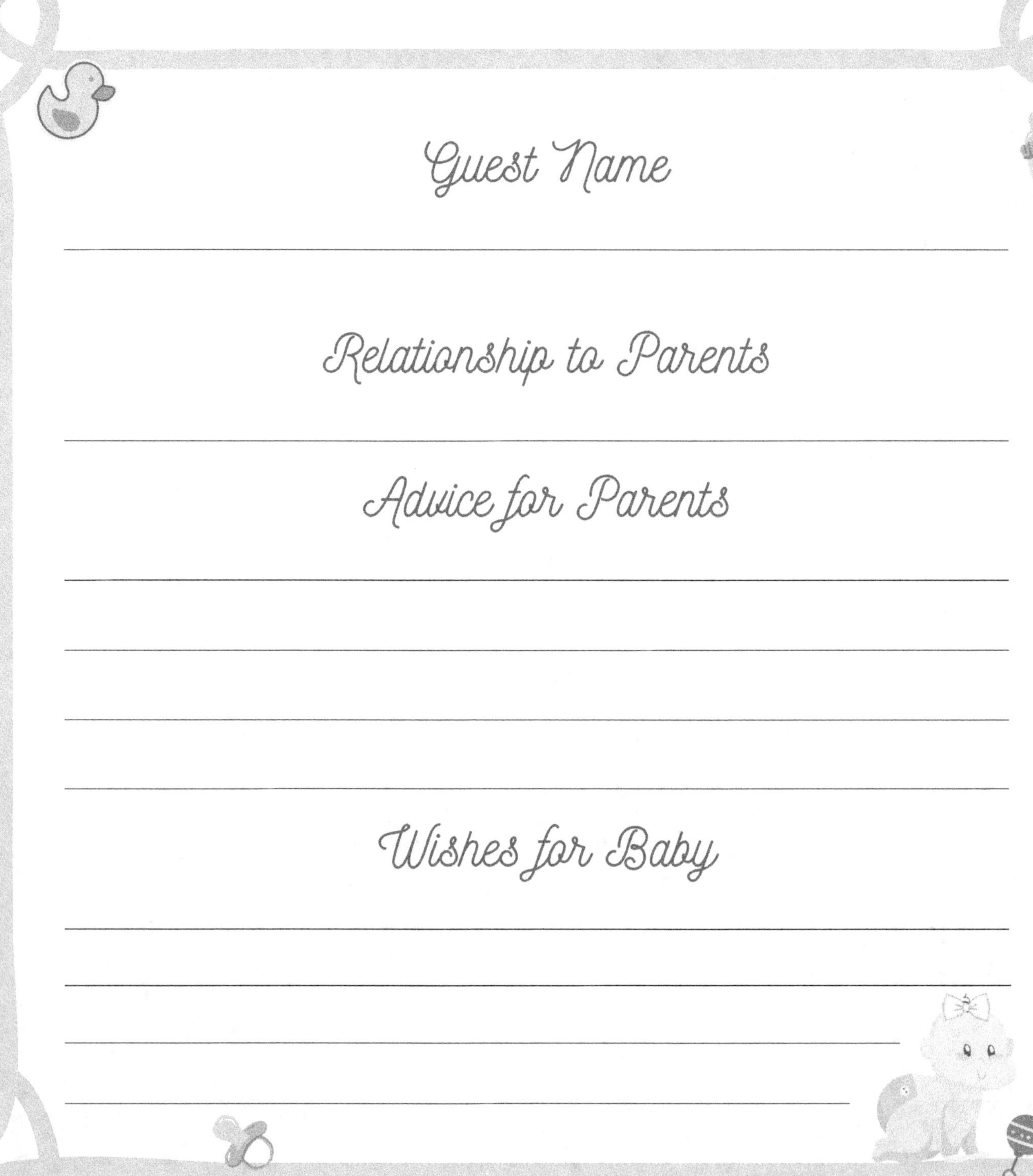

Guest Name

Relationship to Parents

Advice for Parents

Wishes for Baby

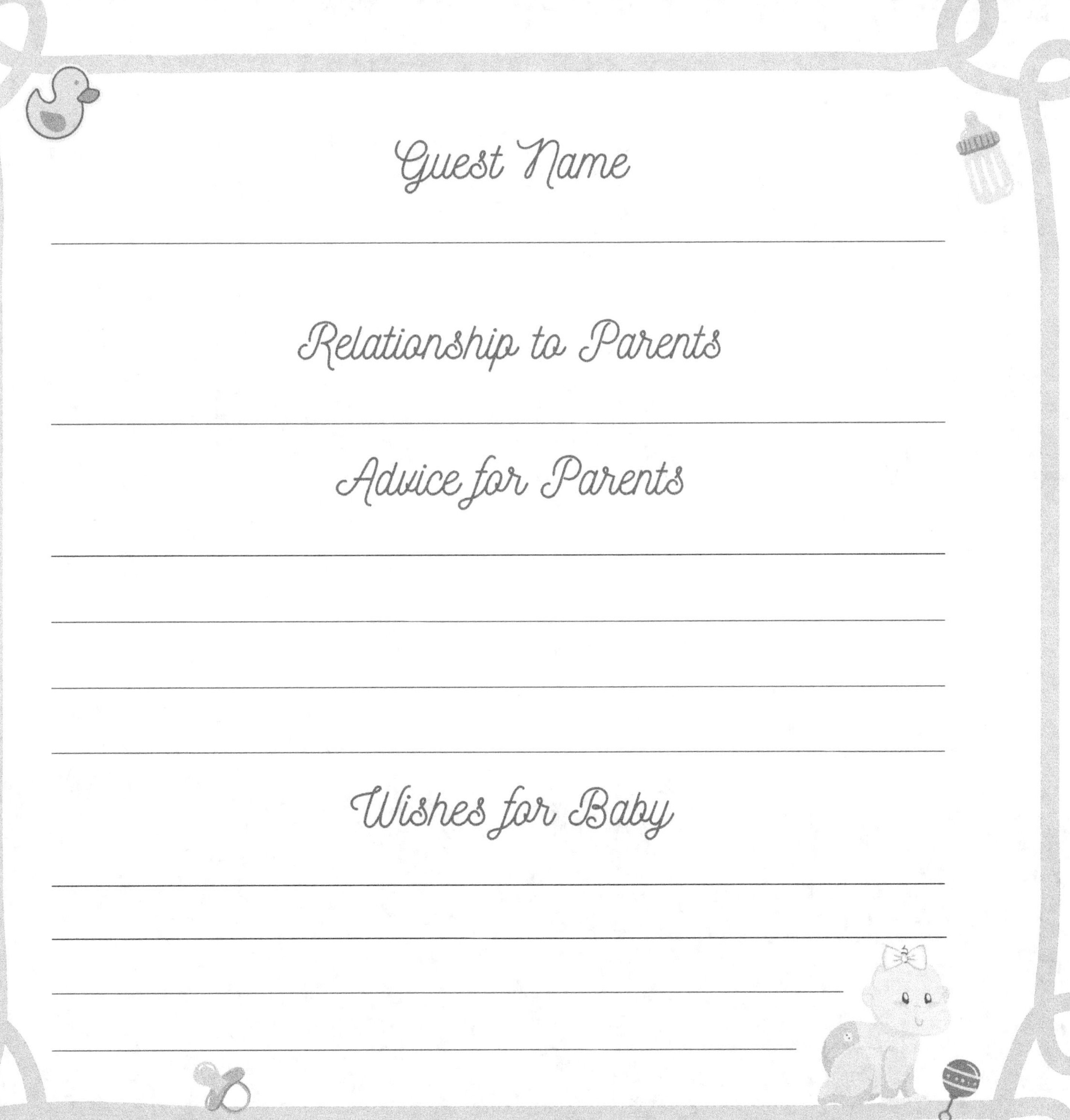

Guest Name

Relationship to Parents

Advice for Parents

Wishes for Baby

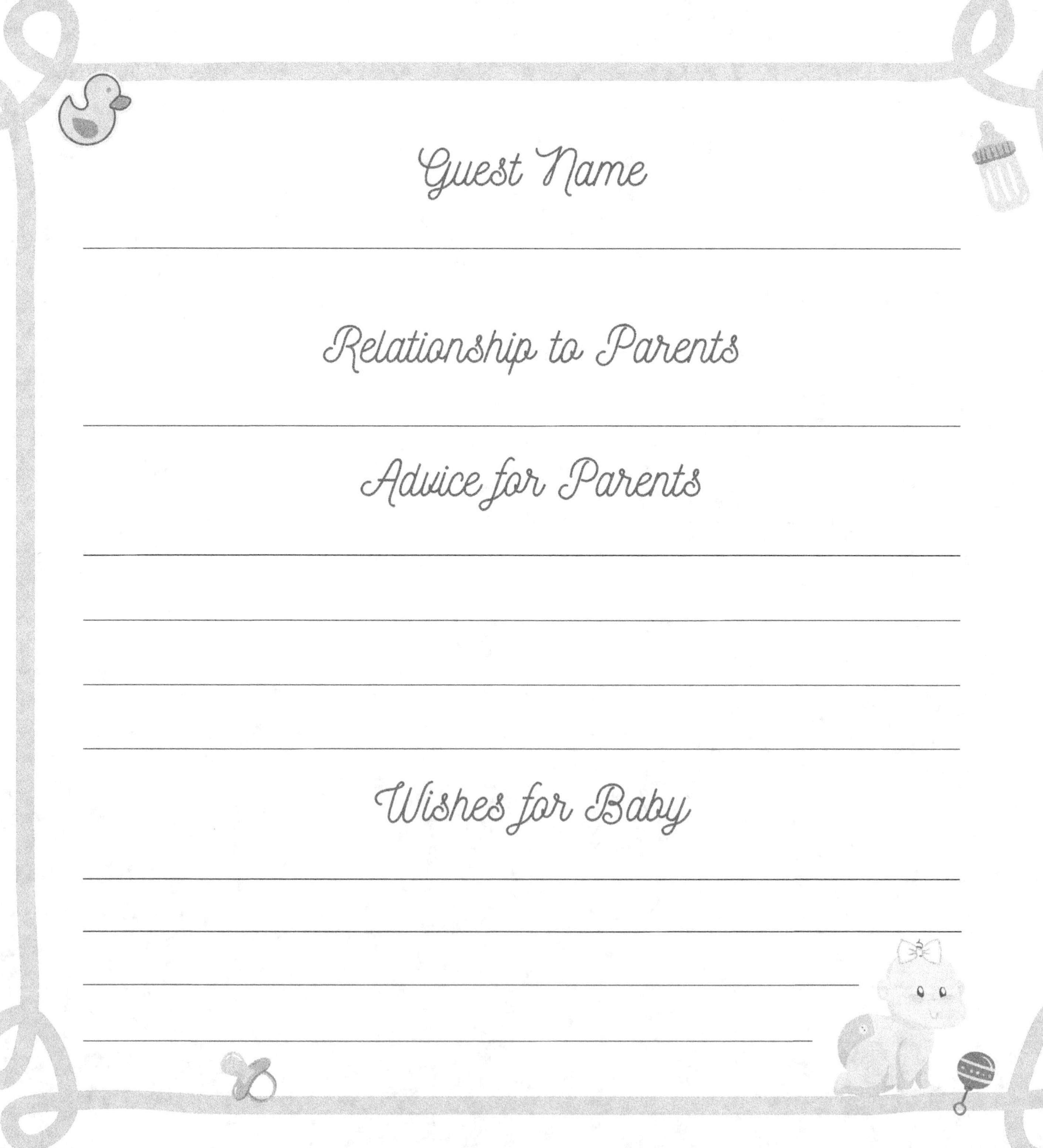
Guest Name
Relationship to Parents
Advice for Parents
Wishes for Baby

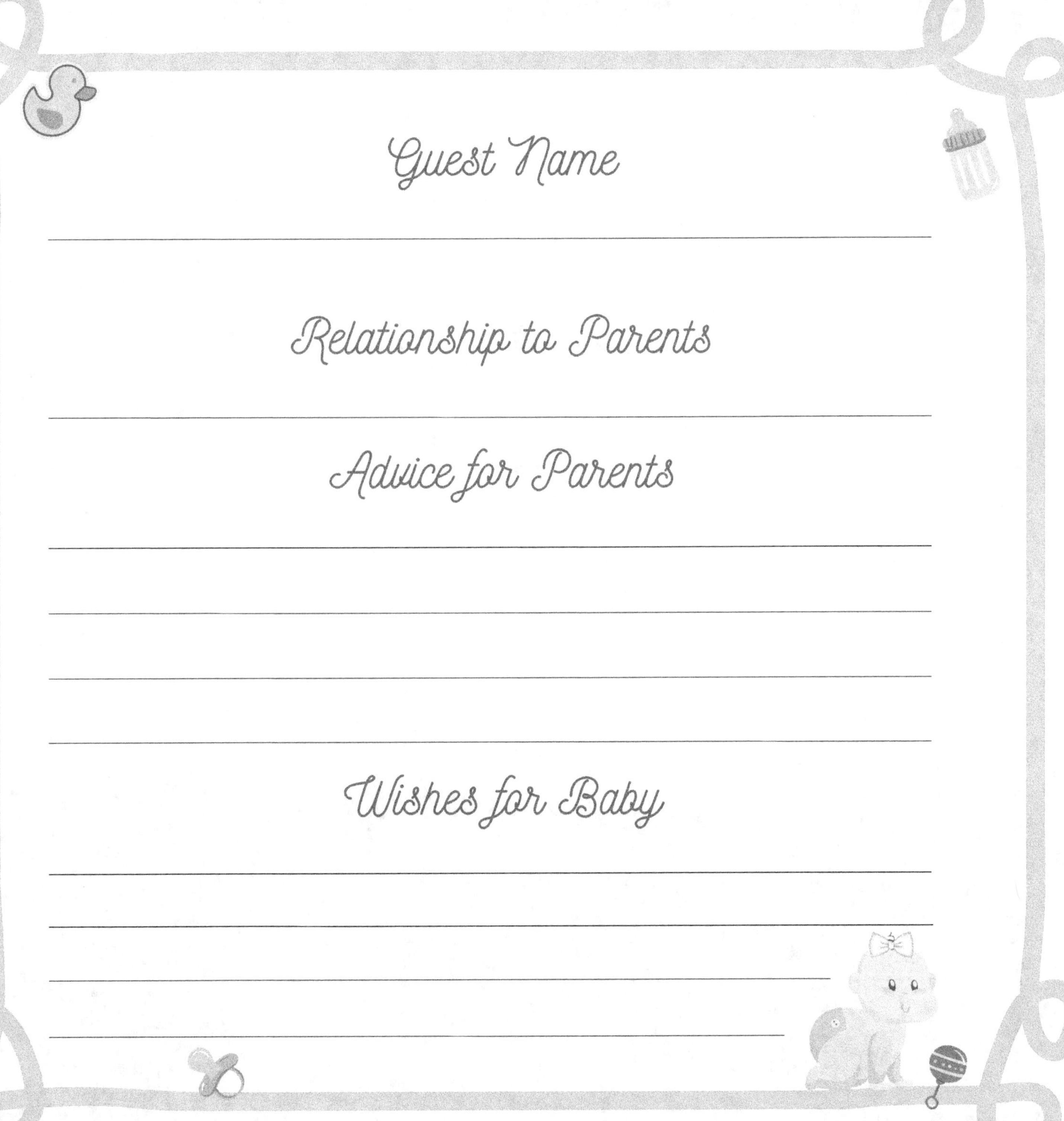

Guest Name
Relationship to Parents
Advice for Parents
Wishes for Baby

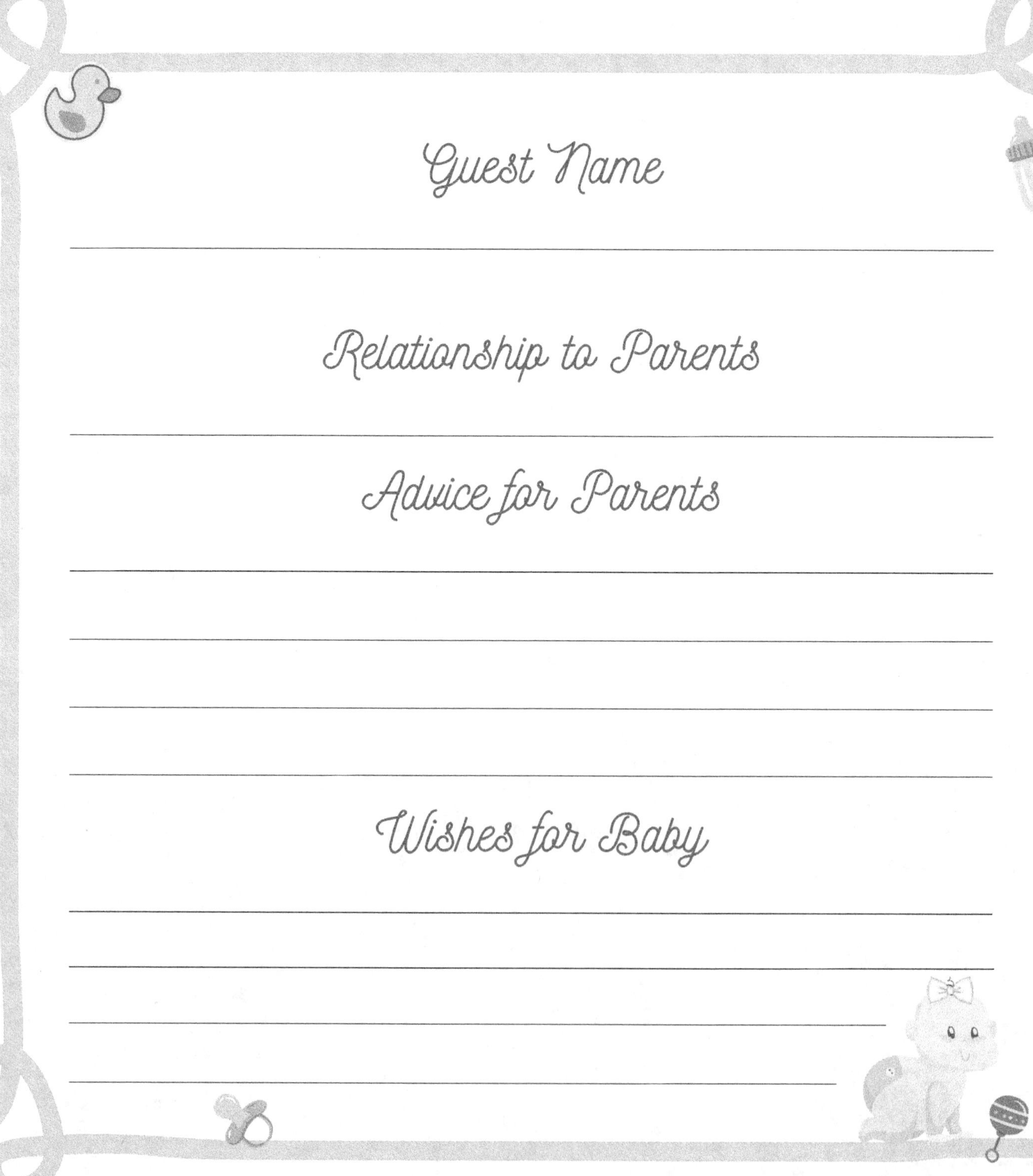

Guest Name

Relationship to Parents

Advice for Parents

Wishes for Baby

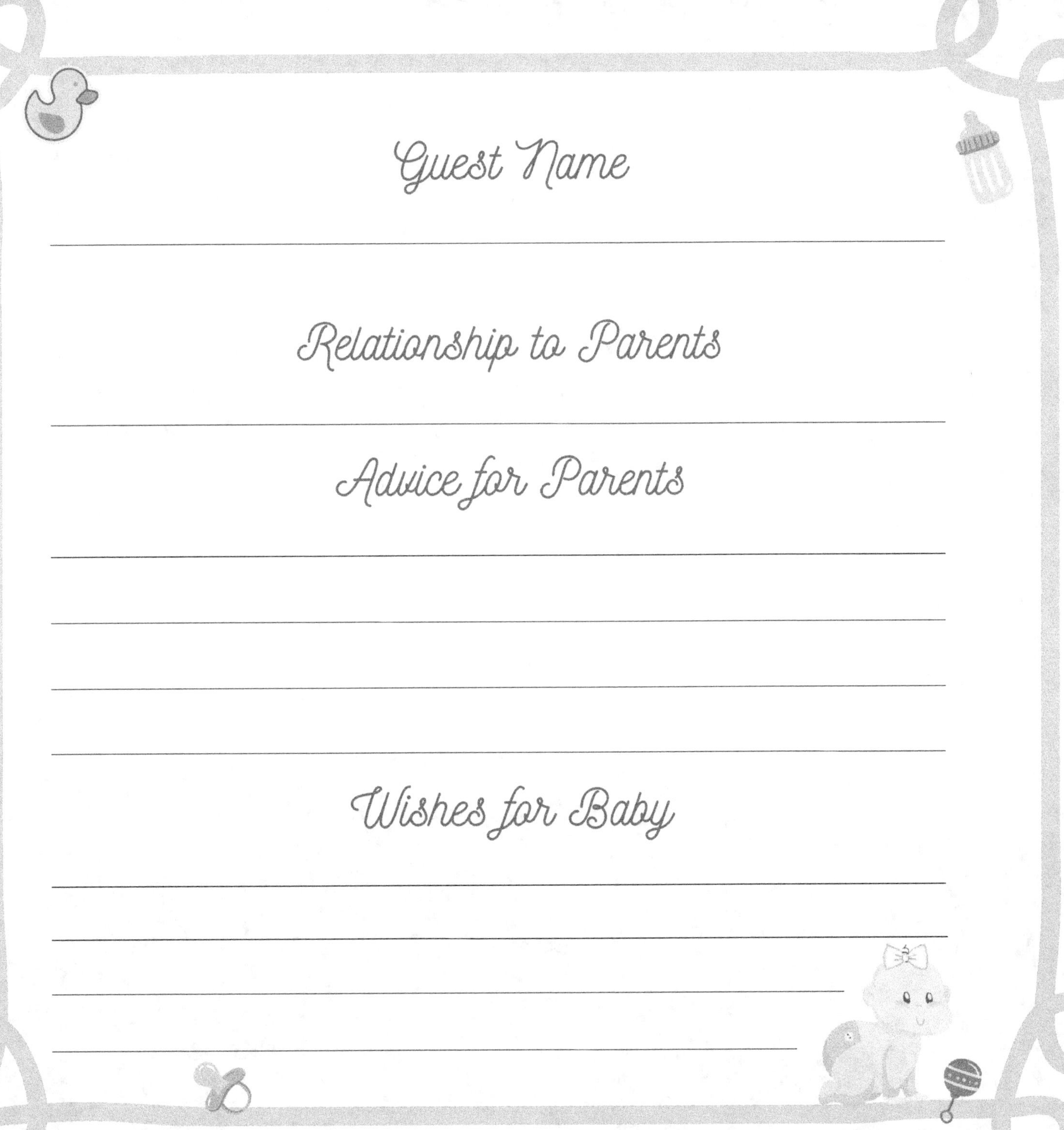

Guest Name
Relationship to Parents
Advice for Parents
Wishes for Baby

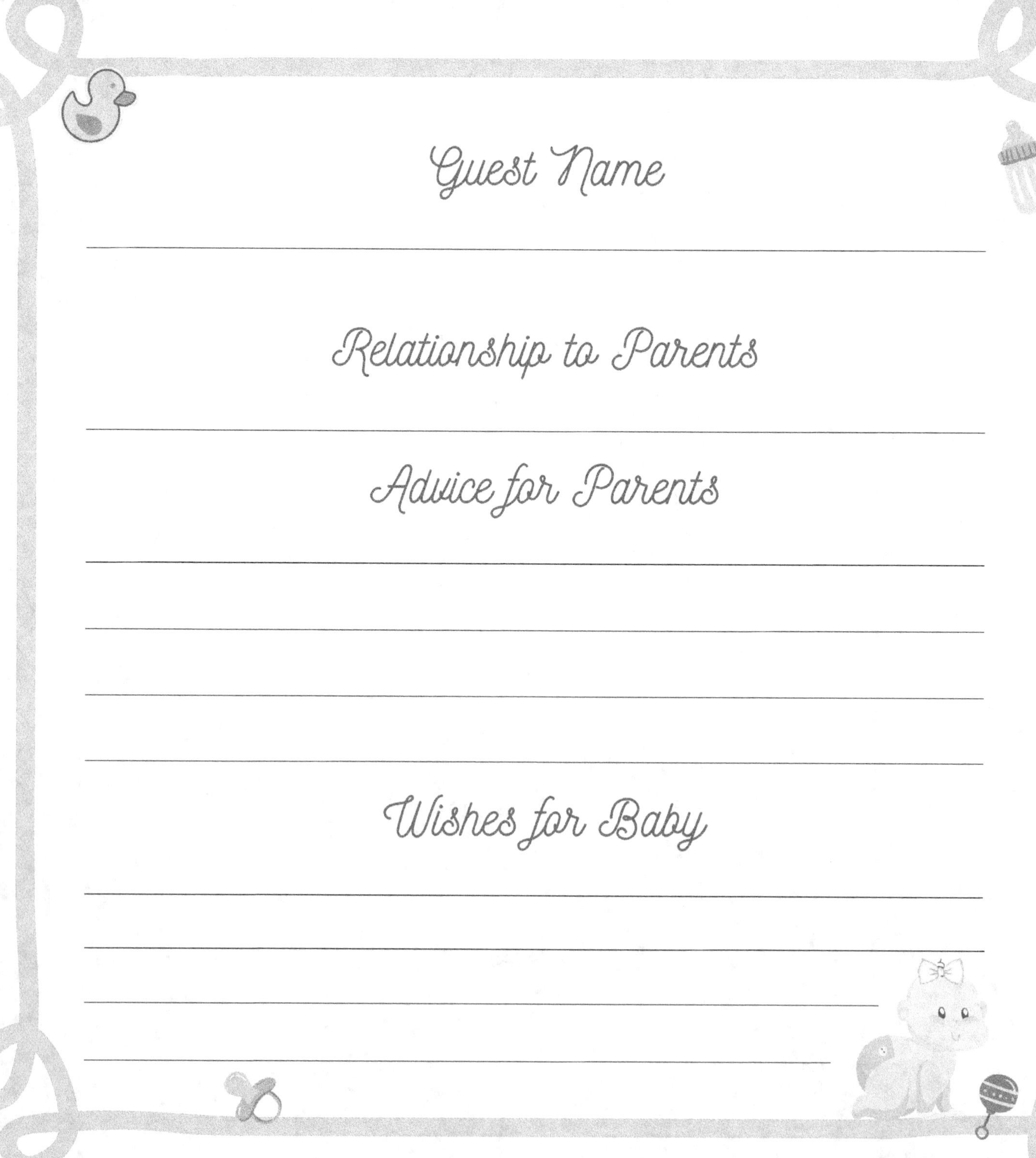
Guest Name

Relationship to Parents

Advice for Parents

Wishes for Baby

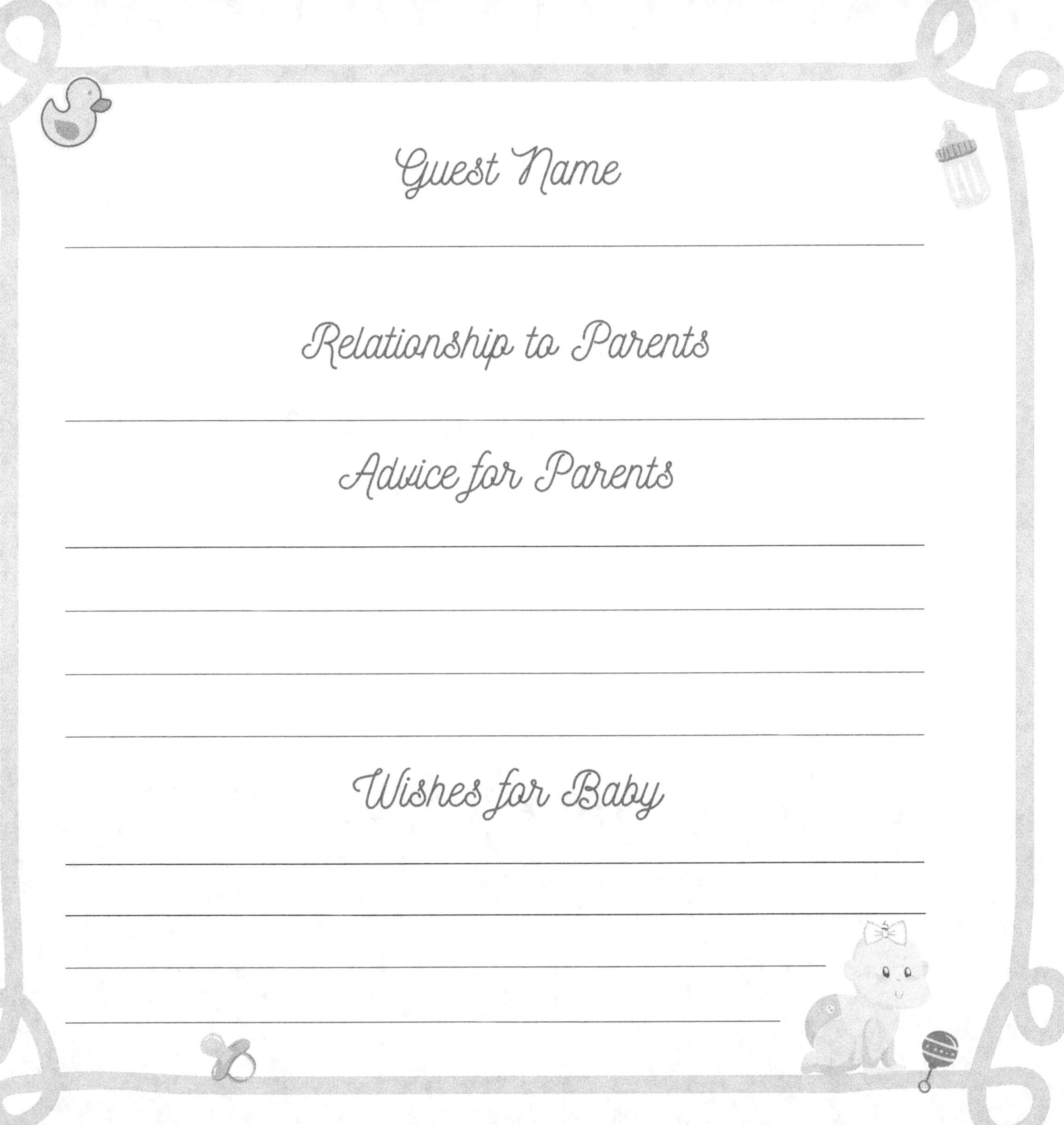

Guest Name
Relationship to Parents
Advice for Parents
Wishes for Baby

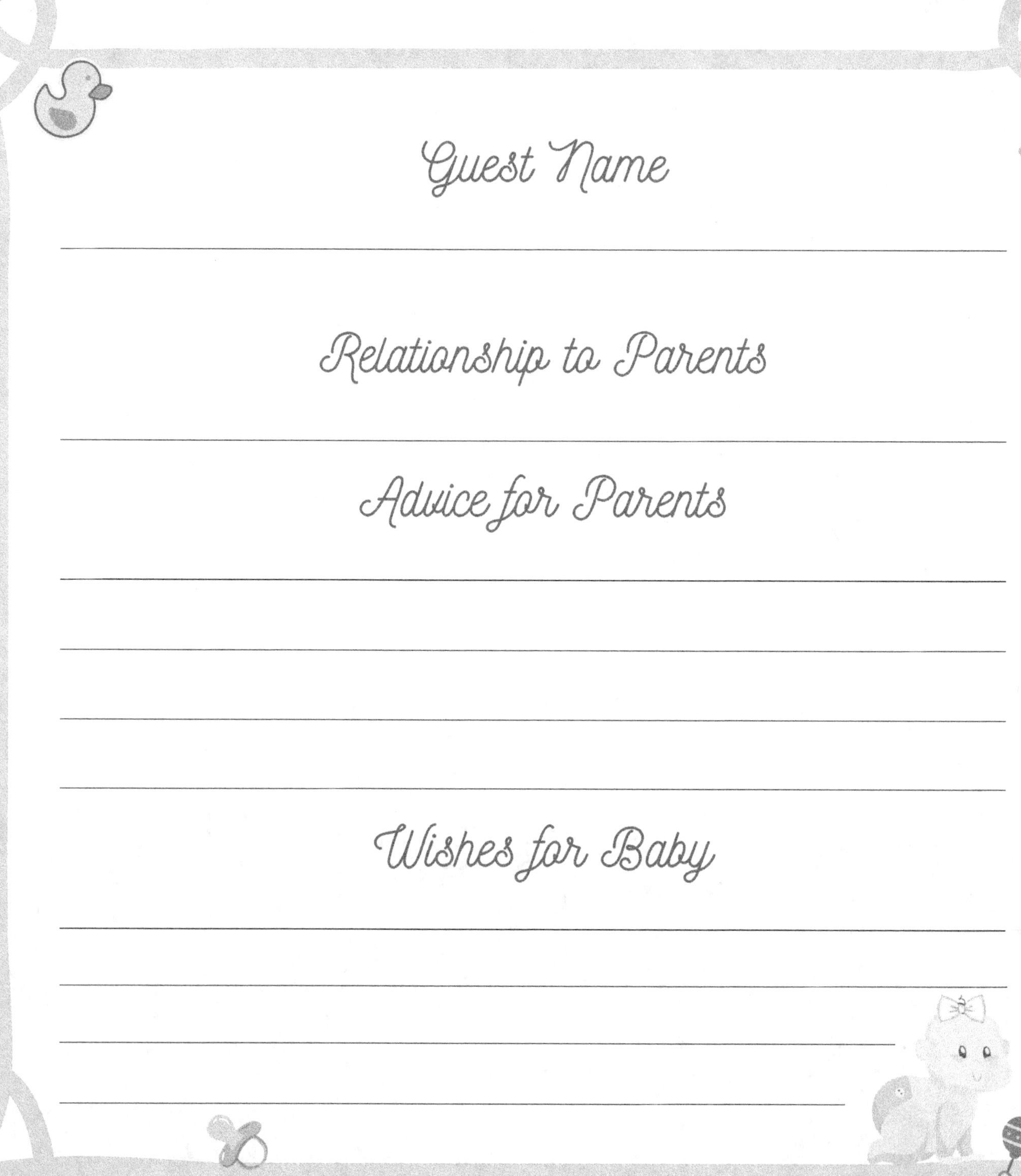

Guest Name

Relationship to Parents

Advice for Parents

Wishes for Baby

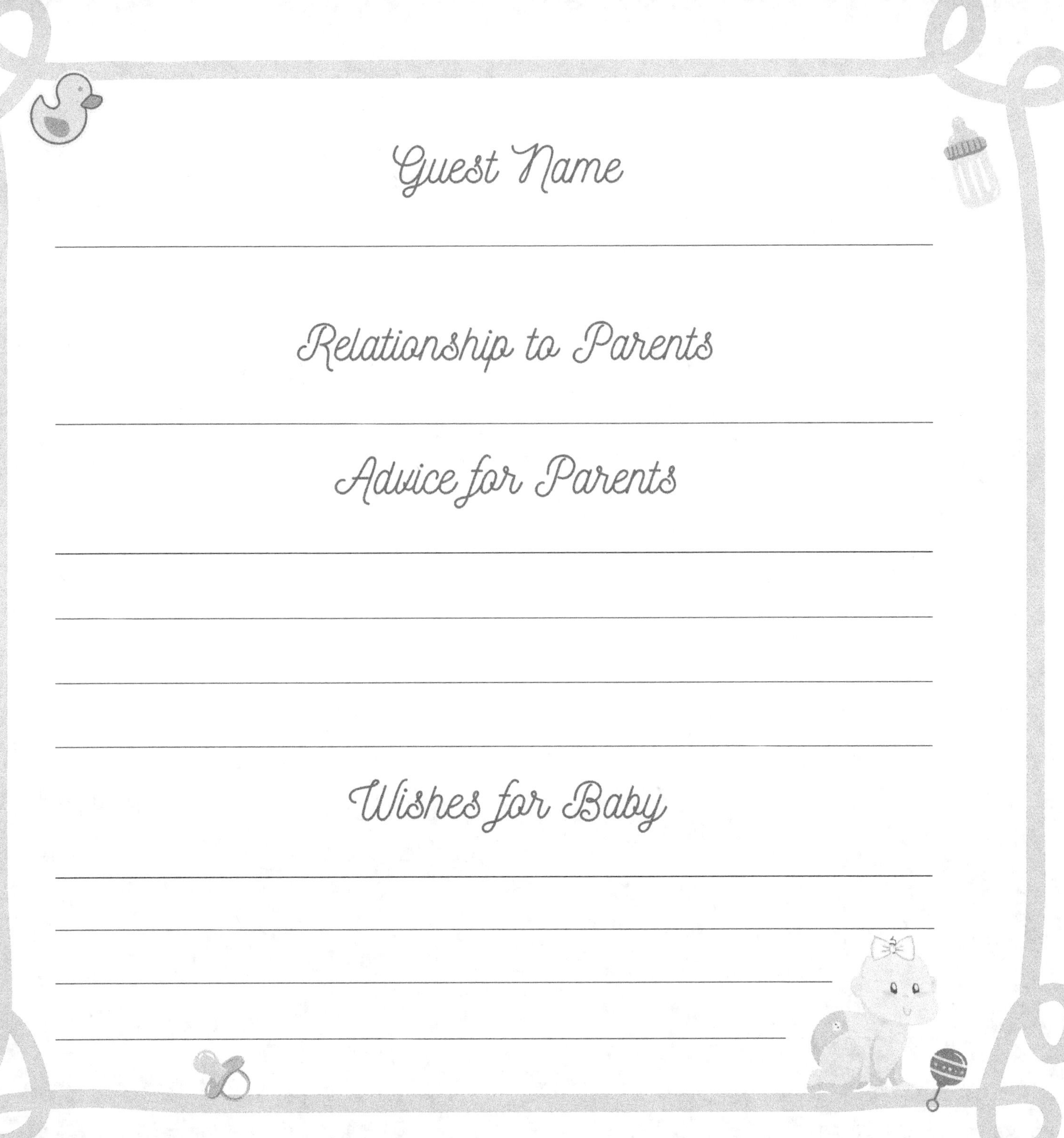

Guest Name

Relationship to Parents

Advice for Parents

Wishes for Baby

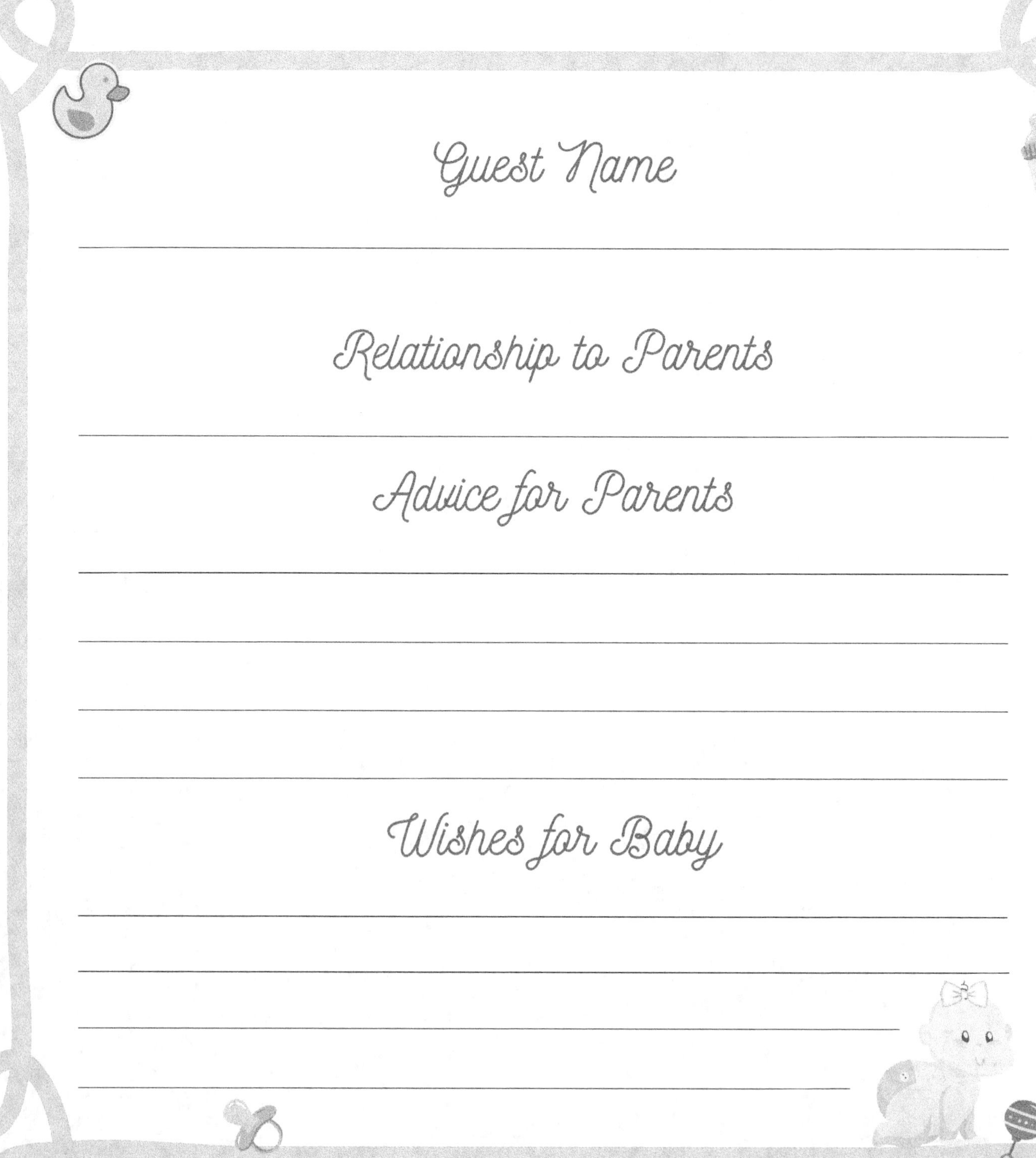

Guest Name

____

Relationship to Parents

____

Advice for Parents

____

____

____

Wishes for Baby

____

____

____

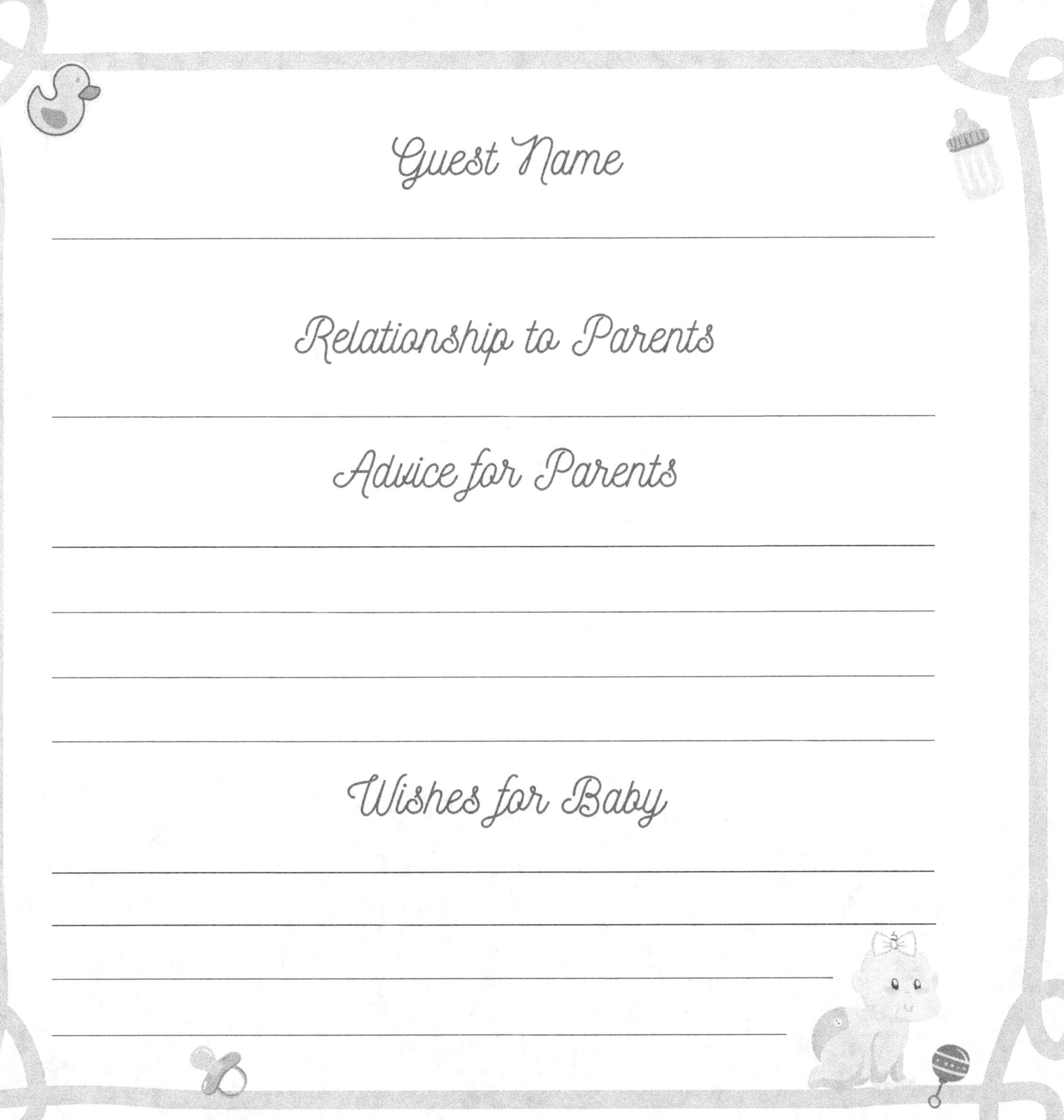

Guest Name

Relationship to Parents

Advice for Parents

Wishes for Baby

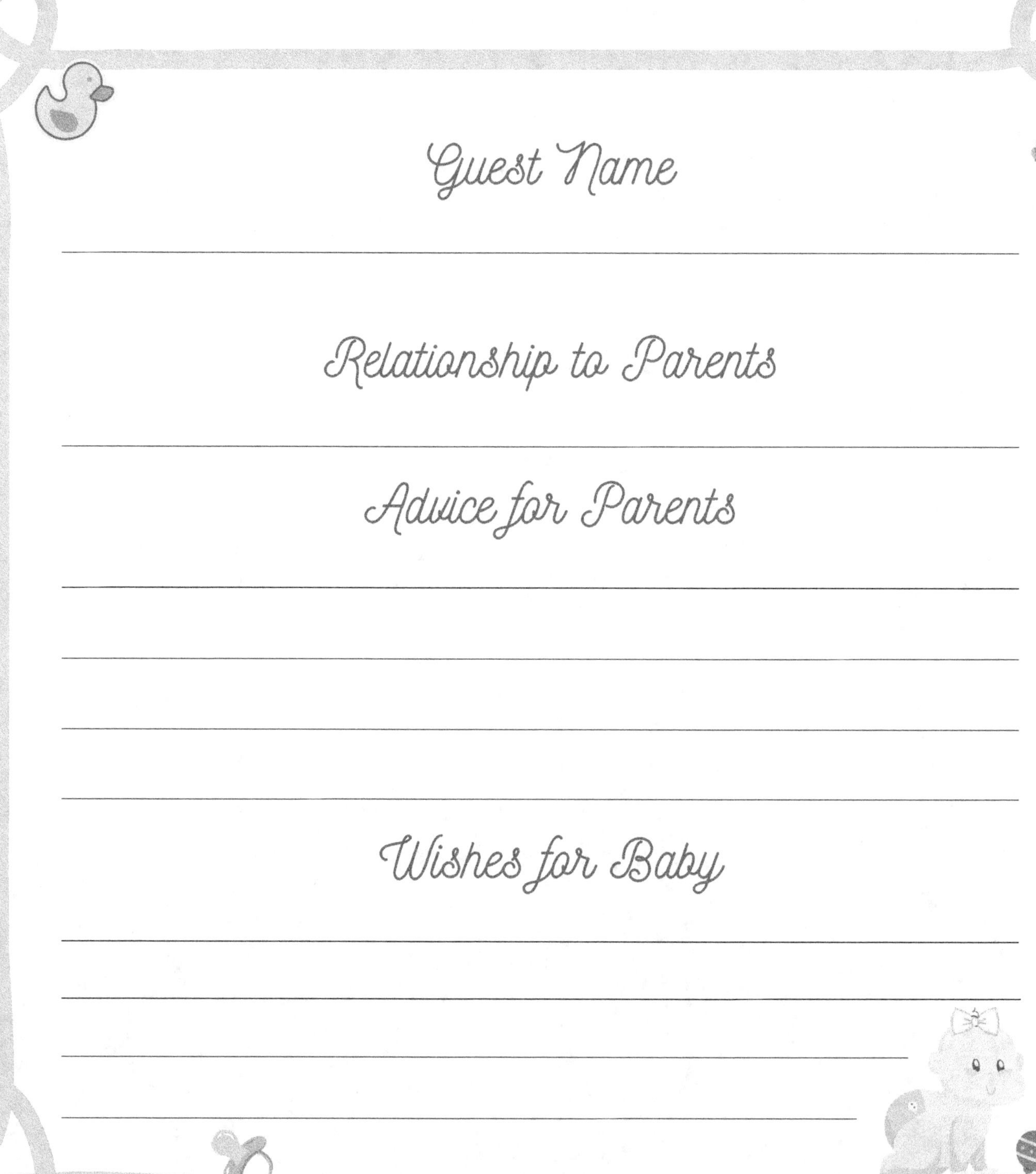

Guest Name
Relationship to Parents
Advice for Parents
Wishes for Baby

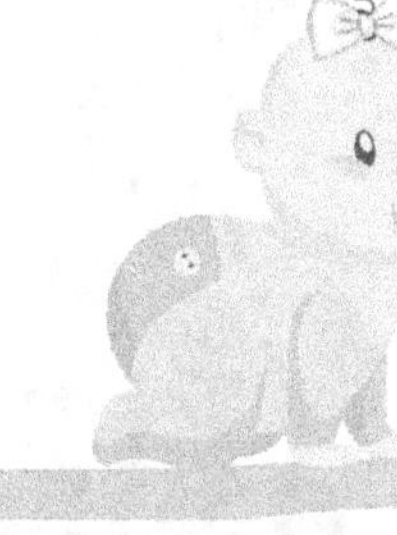
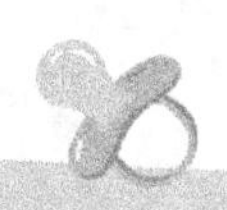

Notes / Photos

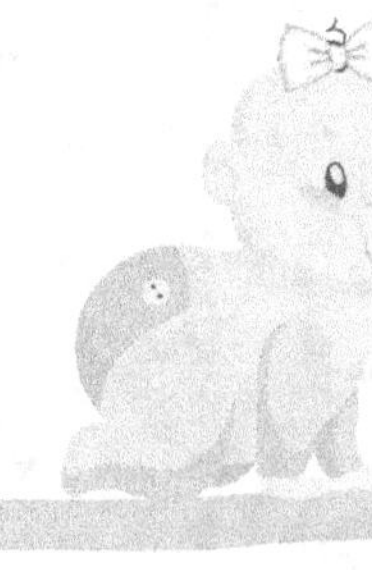
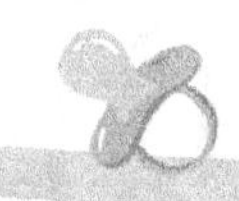

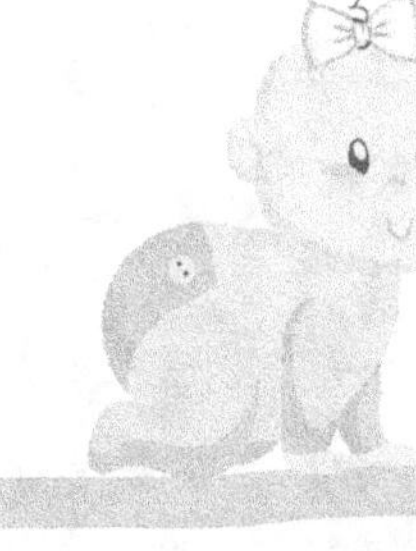

Notes / Photos

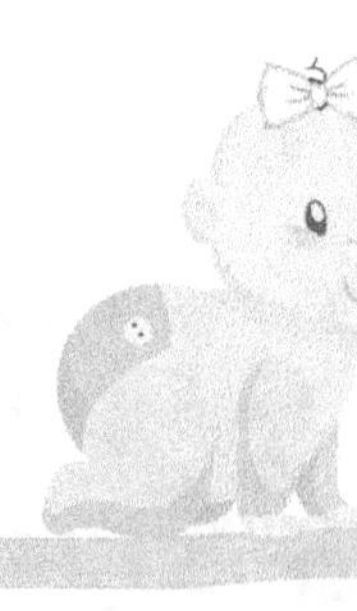
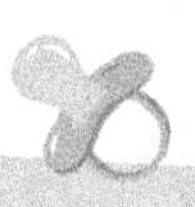

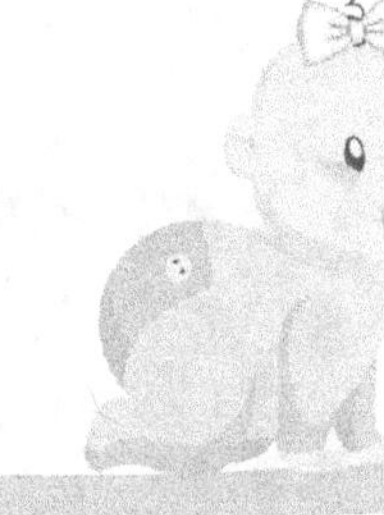

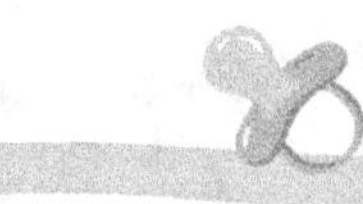

Notes / Photos

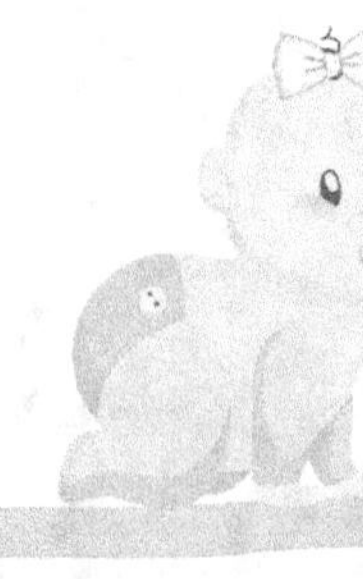
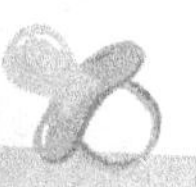

Notes / Photos

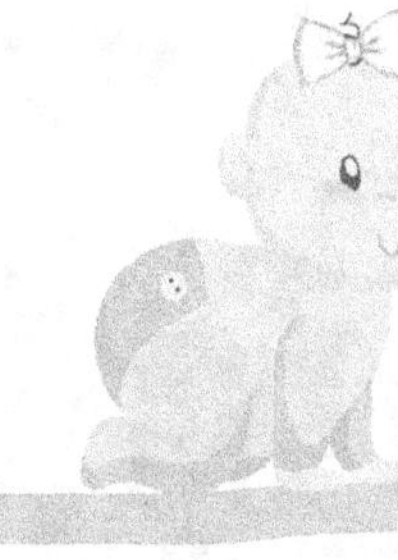

Notes / Photos

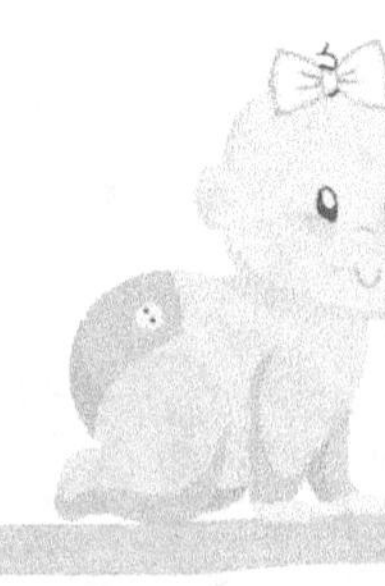
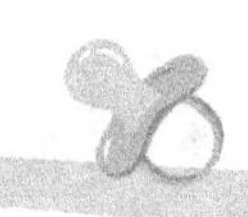

Gift Log

Name/Email/Phone	Gift

Gift Log

Name/Email/Phone	Gift

Gift Log

<table>
<tr><td>*Name/Email/Phone*</td><td>*Gift*</td></tr>
</table>

Gift Log

Name/Email/Phone	Gift

Gift Log

Name/Email/Phone   Gift

Gift Log

Name/Email/Phone	Gift

Gift Log

Name/Email/Phone
Gift

Gift Log

Name/Email/Phone	Gift

Gift Log

Name/Email/Phone   Gift

Gift Log

Name/Email/Phone   Gift

www.ingramcontent.com/pod-product-compliance
Lightning Source LLC
LaVergne TN
LVHW081046210726
843510LV00014B/1047